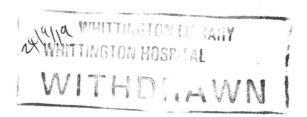
Clinical Supervision for Palliative Care

by
Jean Bayliss

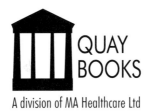

QUAY BOOKS

A division of MA Healthcare Ltd

Quay Books Division, MA Healthcare Ltd, St Jude's Church, Dulwich Road, London
SE24 0PB

British Library Cataloguing-in-Publication Data
A catalogue record is available for this book

© MA Healthcare Limited 2006
ISBN 185642 291 7

Printed in Malta by Gutenberg Press, Gudja Road, Tarxien PLA19, Malta

Contents

Other titles available in the Palliative Care series include:

Aspects of Social Work and Palliative Care
Edited by Jonathan Parker

Counselling Skills in Palliative Care
By Jean Bayliss

Fundamental Aspects of Palliative Care
By Robert Becker and Richard Gamlin

Hidden Aspects of Palliative Care
Edited by Brian Nyatanga and Maxine Astley-Pepper

Palliative Care for the Child with Malignant Disease
Edited by the West Midlands Paediatric Macmillan Team

Palliative Care for People with Learning Disabilities
Edited by Sue Read

Palliative Care for the Primary Care Team
By Eileen Palmer and John Howarth

Palliative Care in Severe Dementia
Edited by Julian Hughes

Palliative Care for South Asians: Muslims, Hindus and Sikhs
Edited by Rashid Gatrad, Erica Brown and Aziz Sheikh

Policy in End-of-Life Care: Education, ethics, practice and research
By Mary Chiarella

Why is it so difficult to die?
By Brian Nyatanga

Work-based Learning in Cancer and Palliative Care
Edited by Liz Searle and Brian Nyatanga

Series Editor: Brian Nyatanga

Note: Health care practice and knowledge are constantly changing and developing as new research and treatments, changes in procedures, drugs and equipment become available. The authors and publishers has, as far as is possible, taken care to confirm that the information in this book complies with the latest standards of practice and legislation.

Introduction

Palliative care is arguably the most stressful area of nursing and care work, as well as being one of the most rewarding. It is an enormous privilege to share the final part of anyone's life journey – a journey that can too often feel lonely – and helping to ease that loneliness as part of a palliative care team is fulfilling and valuable. It is work that requires a high level of practical skill, which can help the dying person to feel more comfortable and confident. But practical skills, valuable though they are, are not enough. Palliative care demands from its practitioners an equally high level of compassion and resilience. Offering this combination of practical comfort and deeply felt concerned support is hugely demanding. Palliative care is a relatively new area of expertise and is growing rapidly, yet in its initial inspiration (and it *was* and *is* inspirational) and in its growth, little consideration has been given to the wants and needs of those who provide the care. Although there is an increasing and welcome realisation that more help is needed for those close to the dying person (those people who we might term 'informal carers' – the relatives and friends) there has been rather less thought given to the wants and needs of the professional carer. Some research has shown that the challenge of providing care at such a profound level can result in the use of 'burn out' and 'distancing' as coping strategies, and it has shown that neither is very desirable. This book is an attempt to suggest a strategy for professional help which will also enhance patient and client care.

Clinical supervision has been researched, promoted, and proven as a very effective strategy for constantly developing skills, for maintaining and raising standards, for encouraging personal and professional development, and for building team ethos. This book therefore explores clinical supervision and the qualities, skills, models and ethics needed to ensure success.

Clinical Supervision for Palliative Care is written as a workbook. You will find pauses for reflection and it is recommended that you keep paper and pen to hand to write down your answers to questions. Good palliative care is based on good communication – so you are asked to interact with the text. The book was researched with a range of professionals working in the field, and with some of those receiving their care. Their experiences are relayed verbatim and with their permission. You will find their words in shaded boxes throughout this book. I am greatly indebted to these people for their time, their frankness and their encouragement – they clearly felt, as I do, that practitioners both need and deserve all the support they can get. I hope that the book will encourage implementation of clinical supervision across the widening field of palliative care – not only because it will support and sustain practitioners (who are not always good at looking after themselves!) But because it will also fulfil the ultimate goal of all of us – the best possible care of dying people, helping them to the death that they want, and easing their suffering and that of those closest to them.

CHAPTER 1

What is clinical supervision?

Defining the concept

This book begins with a conundrum. What is clinical supervision? Indeed, is it possible to define it exactly? So many definitions seem to exist that it is worth looking at a few of them so that we may come to some sort of consensus that will guide or 'ground' us as we work through the ensuing chapters. But first, try to work out your personal definition:

✏ Your thoughts

How would you define supervision?
How would you define clinical supervision?

A dictionary definition will usually tell us that supervision is something like 'directing or watching with authority, the work, proceedings or progress' of something or someone. It is this sense of 'with authority' which has led to some quite serious misapprehensions about supervision in general and about clinical supervision in particular. This misapprehension is summed up by Feltham and Dryden (1994) in this way:

> *Unfortunately the term supervision still carries connotations of managerial oversight and control, mistrust and coercion...*

It is indeed unfortunate that the term can conjure up often unpleasant images of an overseer of some sort, with no reference to what 'vision' (an important half of the whole word) might imply. 'Vision' has much more positive connotations; it implies imaginative ways of looking at things, perhaps a degree of foresight, and maybe even a degree of wisdom. If we accept this definition, then supervision should have these qualities in abundance.

How does your definition of supervision compare so far?

The word 'clinical' adds a further dimension and tends perhaps to medicalise the concept of supervision. Within the nursing/health care professions, practitioners have been urged to attend not only to the physical needs of the people in their care, but also to their 'social, emotional and psychological requirements' (Butterworth and Faugier, 1992). These closer interpersonal exchanges, which are increasingly advocated, bring health care closer to social work, where supervision has long been a norm, and to counselling, where it is mandatory. In both social work and counselling, the term 'supervision' on its own is more usual, but (especially in counselling) the term 'clinical' often precedes it, and this reminds us that clinical supervision is not confined to a health care or medical sphere. As palliative care is often teamwork (it may involve counsellors and social workers) this is important.

So, what are we talking about? What *is* clinical supervision?

Here are some definitions. As you read each one, take time to record how far you agree or disagree with each writer's views – and remember that your own definition has value too.

1. Client-work supervision is a formal process that provides a practitioner with the discipline and support of an experienced colleague in the careful and confidential oversight of the practitioner's work with clients. The supervision relationship is a mutual one and is not in any way hierarchical, nor must it be confused with formal management (COSCA, 1996).

2. Clinical supervision is a practice-focused professional relationship, involving a practitioner reflecting on practice guided by a skilled supervisor (Bishop, 2001).

3. Supervision is a working alliance between a worker or workers, in which the workers can reflect on themselves in their working situation by giving an account of their work, and receiving feedback and, where appropriate, guidance (Proctor, 1988; Inskipp and Proctor, 1989).

4. Supervision is a formal and mutually agreed arrangement; the task is to work together to ensure and develop the efficacy of the supervisee's practice (BACP, 1996).

5. Clinical supervision is an integral, formalised, yet flexible element of professional practice, utilising a range of strategies aimed at facilitating support and development for practitioners whilst also safeguarding standards and upholding 'best practice' in a non-threatening manner (Bishop, 2001).

✎ Your thoughts

Which definitions of clinical supervision do you agree with?
Which definitions of clinical supervision do you disagree with?

Whether you agree or disagree with these definitions, or with part(s) of them, some points seem to stand out particularly clearly. Let's look at some of these points in order:

1. **Clinical supervision is non-hierarchical** although in work terms a supervisor may be higher up the career ladder than a supervisee, when they meet for clinical supervision they meet as equals. This is why, in general terms, it is not recommended that a supervisee's line manager becomes his or her supervisor. One reason for this is that the supervisee might be reluctant to discuss uncertainties with the very person who will conduct an appraisal and who might have some influence over promotion prospects. If you think of yourself as a supervisee or a potential supervisee you can perhaps understand the difficulties posed by hierarchy, however much you might like and respect your line manager. The situation may be especially difficult for voluntary helpers, who may be managed by a professional, and it can be equally difficult for the supervisor of the volunteers! Try to list some other difficulties you can envisage with hierarchy:

2. **Clinical supervision is about work** in this sense it is less about the practitioners themselves and more about their interactions with clients and patients. This is not to say that clinical supervision is not supportive – it is – but it does highlight the fact that it is very different from personal counselling or therapy.

3. **Clinical supervision encourages reflective practice** in the busy world of nursing and care (or of teaching or any other work involving interaction with people), it is too often difficult to find time to reflect on practice and process. Yet research by professional bodies shows it is very clear that reflection raises standards (as well as providing a range of other benefits which we will look at in a later chapter). Reflective practice is a term that has become very popular in nursing, counselling, and care circles. It seems to be used as a term of general approval – reflective practice is A Good Thing – yet too often there is

insufficient time allocated for practitioners to carry out such reflection. A supervisee interviewed on this matter expressed this paradox to me: 'you're supposed to reflect on your practice, but if you try to, you're seen as self-indulgent or something.'. A well implemented system of clinical supervision should aim to remedy this paradox.

4. **Clinical supervision depends upon some sort agreement between the partners in the 'working alliance** this may be anything from a fairly formal contract or agreement, to a more loosely agreed arrangement to meet regularly to focus on the supervisee's work. There is, however, a clear indication that there should be some sort of mutually agreed arrangement to meet regularly. If clinical supervision is haphazard or *ad hoc* it is unlikely to provide the kind of structured reflection which seems so universally approved of.

Bishop's definition (Bishop, 2001) sums up these points, whilst adding that Clinical Supervision is non-threatening, which brings us back to the early part of this chapter where we mentioned that the term can have quite threatening overtones for some people.

If clinical supervision is seen as authoritarian or as disciplinary, it hardly seems likely that it will promote the type of reflective practice so desirable in care work! To ensure the non-threatening nature of supervision requires skill on the part of the supervisor, as well as a willingness on the part of the supervisee to enter into the 'working alliance'.

Look again at the personal definitions you attempted earlier. Would you like to alter or amend them in any way? If so, how? Why? Why not?

✐ Your thoughts

What amendments, if any, would you make to your personal definitions?

If you review the definitions quoted previously, does there seem to you to be anything missing?

✐ Your thoughts

What 'concept' is missing from the quoted definitions?

Is there a sense that there is insufficient emphasis on the client or patient? Clinical supervision could be seen as a triangular dynamic; the supervisor and the supervisee are clearly vital, but the work that they are focused on is (or should be) the client's or patient's welfare – even though he or she may never be known to the supervisor.

We shall be exploring models of clinical supervision in later chapters, but the role of the client or patient in the process is crucial. This point is made not to minimise the importance of the working alliance between supervisor and supervisee – far from it – but to emphasise that they are not the only players in the drama, and (to carry the analogy a little further) that the client or patient may be the lead player or star. This brings us to consider what the functions and benefits of clinical supervision might be.

Functions of clinical supervision

A useful and easily remembered way of looking at clinical supervision is that its functions are:

- Formative
- Normative
- Restorative

Let's look at each of these in turn.

Formative

Continuing professional development (CPD), the advent of post-qualification portfolios of learning and training, the emphasis on evidence-based practice and a growing insistence on accountability, all point towards the need to engage in life-long learning. The formative function of clinical supervision has an important role in this.

Firstly, it can help with skills development. Even health care workers who have recently trained find that the rapid progress of technology or changes in managing patient care can create anxiety about being up to date. These concerns may be a real source of stress for practitioners who trained some time ago, and for those re-entering the health professions after a break – perhaps for child rearing. And the problem is not confined to the health care professions. Here is what a teacher said when he returned to teaching after a spell working in industry.

👁 **Witness statement**

Things had changed so much. I knew nothing about SATs and I nearly drowned in the paperwork. Even in the classroom I felt like an alien – the way I had taught (and been taught myself) was definitely 'out'. There was a lot to learn about the social aspects too – never being alone with a pupil, for instance. I tell you, I could really have done with someone to guide me through all this, in a proper structured way. I just had to pick it up as I went along.

Take a moment to jot down what you think this teacher needed, bearing in mind that as far as his academic subject was concerned, he was probably the most up-to-date member of the staff.

✏ **Your thoughts**

How could this teacher have been helped?

It seems that as well as receiving clear instruction about the paper work, this teacher needed to develop new skills; he needed to re-think his classroom style, and to employ different ways of imparting the knowledge that he certainly had (these are formative functions). He also had to reflect on how to fulfil his pastoral role, while at the same time not breaching school and government regulations about not being alone with a pupil (these are normative functions). It may not be appropriate here to use the word 'clinical' but a degree of supportive supervision would have been very helpful.

Spending time identifying where there might be skill shortages or which skills might need updating leads to reflection and to better practice.

Clients and patients often raise specific issues that relate to practice which can be discussed in (clinical) supervision and thus lead to new understanding. Look at the experience of a midwife (midwives have statutory practice supervision but this was her experience of clinical supervision):

> **👁 Witness statement**
>
> Everything possible had been done, but, sadly, the baby died – it was probably not viable at that early date, but we worked very hard to give it a chance. If I had the time again I don't think I would have done anything differently. What I hadn't expected, and felt at a loss to deal with, was the *father's* grief. We have some training in helping mothers, but I really didn't know how to react. I've talked to some of the others (colleagues) and they say it's a difficulty for them too. I think we really need some training.

The midwife's supervisor was able to help her to locate suitable training, and to rehearse ways of approaching managers for funding and other resources.

> **✐ Your thoughts**
>
> What, in your view, did this clinical supervision provide?

You might have come up with:

- A safe environment to discuss a specific skill deficit.
- An opportunity to explore a possible solution.
- A strategy for putting the solution into practice.

The midwife summed it up in this way:

> **👁 Witness statement**
>
> Without my clinical supervision, nothing would have changed. I'd have just gone on hoping that it didn't happen again – until it did, of course! I'm so much more confident now.

We could see the formative element as a process, as shown below:

Reflection on an experience or on an issue raised by a client
↓
New understanding
↓
Skill development
↓
Enhanced knowledge and increased self-esteem
↓
Improved practice and better patient care

The cycle might then begin again.

Normative

In the health and care professions (and in other professions too) we hear a great deal about standards. Very often there is a strongly negative sense that standards are 'falling' or 'declining'. Take a moment or two to jot down whether you agree or disagree that this is so, and give some examples from as many areas as you can.

✐ Your thoughts

Do you think that standards are falling in the health care profession?

The normative element of clinical supervision is about monitoring standards. It provides an opportunity to consider how work/practice that is (probably) 'good enough' could be made better and matches this to both national and 'agency' standards.

Depending upon your professional area, what are the national standards for your work?

✐ Your thoughts

Which national standards apply to your work?

Do these differ in any way from standards decided by your employing agency, for example a primary care trust (PCT) or local education authority (LEA)? A look at your mission statement might help you.

Sometimes there is a conflict between these two sets of standards; the national standards for access to a cancer specialist, for instance, may differ greatly from local standards across the UK. The media frequently remind us of the so-called 'postcode lottery' where patients in one area may be prescribed drugs while those in another are denied them. Another example is that parents should be able to send children to the school of their choice, but this often proves impossible.

This tension about standards can be very dispiriting for practitioners. Scrutinising standards is, in a sense, an ethical activity. Most, if not all, professions have a code of ethics and practice: for instance, the British Association for Counselling and Psychotherapy (BACP) have their own code *Ethical Framework for Good Practice in Counselling and Psychotherapy* (BACP, 2001), and nurses have the NMC (formerly the UKCC). If we have an ethical dilemma, it should be possible to get help by referring to our professional codes. What then do you think of this comment, made by a well known writer on supervision (Carroll, 1996):

> *Ethical codes do not give answers to many individual situations, and it is here that clinical supervision can provide the forum that alerts to ethical sensitivity and allows for reflection preceding decisions.*

Carroll seems to be saying that although our professional codes may be useful, when we have a personal ethical dilemma we need clinical supervision in order to sharpen up our ethical awareness, and that this should help with decision making about practice. Carroll also conveys the sense that if clinical supervision is in place there is a structure for considering ethical issues *before* we make decisions, as well as reflecting on ethical decisions after the event. Clinical supervision's normative function therefore has a preventative role.

Read the following witness statement (made specifically for this book by a district/community nurse, who was working with a hospice-at-home team and visiting a palliative care patient):

◉ Witness statement

When it got to the weekend it was obvious that the end was very near. She had no close relatives near (her only child is in New Zealand) and she had told me that she had made an advance directive that she should be 'allowed to go', as she put it. (I think now that I was the only person who knew about that.) On my morning visit she was comfortable but frail and told me that a friend was calling later. When I went in the late afternoon she had died and it was evident she had used the diamorphine (which was out of her reach) to hasten her end. My guess is that she had asked the friend to put the medication within reach without telling her what it was, although of course I can't actually know that. I just didn't know what to do: there seemed little point in a post-mortem as she was near the end anyway. If I said anything about the moving of the medication it could implicate the friend and perhaps leave her with a load of guilt. I also didn't know whether to put the medication back where it had been.

Now jot down what your own decision might have been, and how you think clinical supervision might have helped.

✐ Your thoughts

What would your ethical decision have been? What are your reasons?
Would reference to your code of ethics have helped? Why?
How might clinical supervision have helped?

In recent years, professionals have become used to targets. Some practitioners find the targets irksome and not always in the best interest of the client or patient. In one survey an anonymous doctor was quoted as saying:

◉ Witness statement

It's ridiculous! We have this target that no one waits in A&E for more than four hours. So what happens? Patients stay in ambulances outside the hospital or wait around so that admission time gets pushed back. Then they're seen but no treatment may be given, so they're left on trolleys.

As you can tell, he was very angry. What these targets do not seem to do, even if they are met, is measure the quality of practice, and this applies to many areas, not only to A&E departments in hospitals. In the busy and often hectic rush of day-to-day practice it is not easy to stand back and reflect on whether things could be (or should be) done differently, or on how to go about changing things if necessary. Indeed, change is in itself stressful and perhaps clinical supervision has an important ethical role here. If you look back over an average week or month of your working pattern, how often have you had the opportunity to reflect on the quality of your own practice, and, if you have a responsibility for managing others, to consider their practice?

✐ **Your thoughts**

How often have you reflected on the quality of your own practice?
Have you reflected on the practice of people who work for you?

Malpractice and 'just about passable' practice are usually easy to spot (not always so easy to remedy!) But measuring 'good enough' practice against national or local norms too often gets crowded out.

There has been a noticeable increase in the use of questionnaires and feedback forms. Clients and patients are asked to fill these in 'so that we can improve our service to you'. This process can be a very valuable agent for change, but only if that feedback is considered and acted on. Unfortunately, all too often those forms are filed, possibly because no consensus can be reached as to how best to act on the feedback. This can lead to cynicism – a very negative state. A recent Ofsted (Office for Standards in Education) inspection observed that one particular school's staff seemed very stressed, and they recommended that some help be given to alleviate this. A half-day's training in stress management was arranged, but only a few staff members turned up, one of whom confided to the trainer that the appropriate box could now be ticked and staff could no longer be stressed! A similar degree of cynicism can result from many such 'initiatives'. Good, structured clinical supervision can help to minimise disillusionment, as well as help to monitor standards.

There is increasing emphasis on the need for **accountable practice.** In most, if not all, professions the practitioner's responsibility is increasingly highlighted. So whilst poor practice is evident, measuring the quality of day-to-day accepted practice often doesn't happen. Opportunities to improve it may then be lost (and sadly, sometimes never again looked at).

✏ **Your thoughts**

To whom do you feel responsible?
For whom do you feel responsible?

The normative element of clinical supervision can well be seen as an instrument for quality control and it is certainly a vehicle for promoting and maintaining standards.

Read again the witness statement of the district nurse with the ethical dilemma; as this brings us to the third element of clinical supervision – the restorative.

Restorative

If we work with people, especially people who are stressed by illness or other concerns, it is inevitable that we will ourselves experience some level of work-related stress. The restorative element of clinical supervision can help with this, as long as the boundary between restorative supervision and personal counselling or therapy is clear and is firmly maintained. A practitioner may well benefit from personal counselling, and this may become evident during clinical supervision, but if so a referral to a more appropriate form of help should be negotiated. Even so, the safe forum provided by clinical supervision to 'off load' has great value. It is different from what has been called 'tea-break; tear-break' – the sort of mutual support between colleagues who offer each other a 'shoulder to cry on', so to speak. Such mutual care and support is invaluable, but it can be *ad hoc*, and it offers more of a 'safety valve' than a structured time that looks at the causes of the stresses affecting the practitioner's work and which tries to explore strategies for reducing them.

At a recent training event, the group of trainees (thirty of them, plus health professionals) was asked how many people (other than patients/clients) had they praised in the previous week? And how many people had praised them? Sadly, the response to both questions was 'very few'. Ask yourself the same two questions.

✐ Your thoughts

How many people (other than patients/clients) have you praised in the previous week?
How many people have praised you?

As long ago as 1851 John Ruskin (Ruskin, 1871) suggested that:

> *In order that people may be happy in their work, these things are needed:*
>
> *They must be fit for it.*
> *They must not do too much of it.*
> *They must have a sense of success in it.*

✐ Your thoughts

What do you understand by being 'fit' for work?

Obviously, physical fitness is important, but we also need to be fit in other senses too. We need to be 'fit for purpose' which means that not only do we have appropriate training and skills, but also we are not too stressed to do the work well, and (perhaps most important of all) that we are emotionally fit. We can only be fit in all these ways if we keep a sensible work–life balance. Hard-working and dedicated professionals are notorious for over-working, so a supervisor who can point out the danger signs is invaluable for helping to keep the balance.

Lastly, the **restorative** element of clinical supervision can help to fulfil Ruskin's final point – it is the perfect forum for validating and celebrating success.

Formative, normative and restorative are the three most usually stated elements of supervision, but recently an additional element has been added. Review the work you have done so far and try to list anything that you think is missing.

✏ **Your thoughts**

What, if anything, is missing from these elements of Supervision?

The additional element that has been suggested is: **perspective**. There has been a great growth, in virtually all professional areas, of teamworking. If palliative care is taken as an example, can you list the likely members of the team providing the palliative care?

✏ **Your thoughts**

Which people should be on a team that provides palliative care?

You might have mentioned any of these:

- doctors
- hospice nurses
- community nurses
- social workers
- informal carers
- counsellors
- Macmillan nurses/Marie Curie nurses
- care assistants
- pharmacists
- family and volunteer helpers.

Perspective?

The variety of values and expertise in a team can vary enormously – of course this can be enriching, but it can also lead to conflict. Clinical supervision has an important role in developing perspective. The relationship between one's own care expertise and other methods or strategies for client benefit can be usefully explored in supervision, especially if there is conflict. Relationships with other professionals, insight into their ways of looking at a client or patient, and their ways of approaching the work within the 'umbrella' of the team ethos, can be enlightening. Here are witness statements of two members of a palliative care team, who had joint clinical supervision:

◉ Witness statement

Nurse I spent most of the time trying to make the patient comfortable and explaining the syringe driver and medication to the husband, as well as to her. She seemed quite restless and even agitated whatever I did and I wasn't really sure why.

Counsellor I have no real nursing skills, except of the most rudimentary kind, so I tried to help with the agitation. It turned out that she had had a year-long rift with her brother and wanted to put that right before her death.

Both agreed that clinical supervision had helped them to broaden their perspective about different ways of helping the same patient. They went on to reflect how the experience had developed their appreciation of team working and (they joked) 'even team members we don't really like!'.

This chapter began by asking what clinical supervision is, and went on to explore four areas:

- Formative
- Normative
- Restorative
- Perspective

The NMC (former UKCC) position sums up these functions very well (UKCC, 2001):

> *Clinical supervision can help you to develop your skills and knowledge throughout your career. It is an integral part of lifelong learning... Enabling you constantly to evaluate and improve your contribution to patient and client care. Clinical supervision aims to bring practitioners and skilled supervisors together to reflect on practice, to identify solutions to problems, to increase understanding of professional issues and, most importantly, to improve standards of care.*

As a final exercise try to list what you now see as the potential benefits of clinical supervision. (We shall return to this topic later and look at some of the research evidence about benefits.)

✐ **Your thoughts**

What are the benefits to practitioners?
What are the benefits to the organisation?
What are the benefits to clients/patients?

To consolidate your learning from this chapter, try to come up with some answers to the following questions:

✐ **Your thoughts**

In what ways has the term 'supervision' (or clinical supervision) led to a misunderstanding of the functions of clinical supervision?
Can you devise your own definition of each of the four functions of clinical supervision?
Which of the four functions do you see as most beneficial to your own professional area of work? In what way would it be helpful?
Do you agree that clinical supervision should be non-hierarchical? What are your reasons?
What do you see as the obstacles to implementing clinical supervision in your organisation?

References

BACP (1996) *Code of Ethics and Practice for Supervisors of Counsellors.* British Association for Counselling and Psychotherapy, Rugby.

BACP (2001) *Ethical Framework for Good Practice in Counselling and Psychotherapy.* Published by BACP, Rugby

Bishop V (2001) *Fitness for Practice.* UKCC, London

Butterworth T, Faugier J (1992) *Clinical Supervision and Mentoring in Nursing*, 1st edn. Chapman and Hall, London

Carroll M (1996) *Counselling Supervision: Theory, Skills and Practice.* Cassell, London

COSCA (1996) *Statement of Ethics and Code of Practice.* Counselling and Psychotherapy in Scotland, Stirling

Feltham C, Dryden W (1994) *Developing Counsellor Supervision.* Sage Publications, London

Inskipp F, Proctor B (1989) *Skills for Supervisees and Skills for Supervisors* (audiotapes). Alexia Publications, East Sussex

Proctor B (1988) *Supervision: A Working Alliance* (videotape training manual). Alexia Publications, East Sussex

Proctor B (1991) Supervision: a co-operative exercise in accountability. In: Marken M, Payne M (eds) *Enabling and Ensuring Supervision in Practice.* National Youth Bureau, Leicester

Ruskin (1871) *Sesame and Lilies.* HM Caldwell, New York

UKCC (2001) *Supplying nurses, midwives and health visitors through life-long learning.* UKCC Publications

CHAPTER 2

Roles and responsibilities

In *Chapter One* you briefly considered for whom and to whom you felt responsible in your palliative care role. Remind yourself of what your thoughts were.

✐ Your thoughts

For whom and to whom do you feel responsible in your palliative care?

In the working alliance of clinical supervision both parties have a role and a range of responsibilities. These responsibilities are not only to each other, but also to the patients and clients who are 'present' in that relationship, albeit not physically present. When we think about the roles and responsibilities of the supervisor and the supervisee(s), we need to keep this shadowy third person in mind, as the whole point of clinical supervision is to facilitate better patient and client care and to improve the service we offer.

The supervisor

If the working alliance is to be successful, it is evident that both parties will need a range of qualities and skills. We look at the skills of a supervisor in a later chapter, but here let's try to look at what qualities a supervisor might need in order to fulfil the functions we looked at in *Chapter One*.

First, try to list the qualities you yourself would be looking for in a supervisor and then reflect on the extent to which you think you possess them;

✏ **Your thoughts**

What do the ideal qualities of a supervisor include?

Mark on the scale below the extent to which you possess those skills:

[0 ——————————————————————— 100]

For example:

[0 ——————————————————————— 100]

Trust

This list from Butterworth and Faugier (1992) suggests what qualities would be required in a supervisor. This is what they think a supervisor should be:

- generous
- rewarding
- open
- willing to learn
- thoughtful and thought-provoking
- humane
- sensitive
- uncompromising
- good interpersonally
- practical
- trustworthy.

How much does their list agree with yours?

At a recent meeting of would-be clinical supervisors, some interesting suggestions were made for additions to the Butterworth and Faugier list.

They suggested that the supervisor should have some insight into the work under consideration. There was considerable debate about this addition, with wide differences of opinion. At one end of the spectrum, some delegates felt that a supervisor who did not do the same kind of work as their supervisee(s) could not understand the nature of the challenges and stresses the work presented; at the other end were those who thought that reflective practice is better served if the supervisee has to explain interventions to someone from a different discipline (as long as they were not too removed from palliative care) because this made them question their practice more.

✐ Your thoughts

Where would you put yourself on this spectrum?

Supervisor should do the same kind of work as their supervisees

_____

Supervisors should do different work from their supervisees

The ways in which this can affect the working alliance are illustrated by the following two experiences – both are my own, firstly as a supervisee and secondly as a supervisor.

◉ Witness statements

As a supervisee

The supervisor for my counselling practice and I operated from the same theoretical base. I found this quite congenial and even 'cosy' because I could use a sort of 'shorthand' in case discussion. If I referred to universal unconscious or archetype or animus/anima or any of the other terms used in our theoretical orientation, I could be confident that he knew what I was talking about. The shared language certainly meant that we could cover quite a lot of ground in a short time. Then came a time when working with a client from this base just did not seem to work. I felt that I was growing 'stale' and that my skills did not seem to be helping the client to move forward. In retrospect, what I needed was 'prodding' to look at the client in a different way and to review the skills I was using from a different perspective, that is from the *client's* perspective. A supervisor from a different orientation might have 'prodded' me to think differently, which in turn would have made a difference to what skills I was using.

As a supervisor

As a supervisor I have very limited knowledge of nurse/medical interventions except those that I have learned from nurse supervisees. I am therefore able to

cont../.

> Ask 'why did you do that?' or 'what was that intervention intended to achieve?' without in any way questioning the rights or wrongs of an intervention. These questions coming from a fellow nurse practitioner might well be seen as threatening; they might cause offence and result in defensiveness. But because the queries came from someone who genuinely doesn't know the answers and who would like to learn (me – as the supervisor), the supervisee is in a position to define and explain. This in turn helps her to reflect on her own practice and to ask *herself* the question 'Yes, why did I do it that way?'.

So there may be something to be said for both positions, and each alliance will need to decide its own position (and limited availability may mean that there is little choice), but being aware of how this issue affects the dynamic between the participants is critical to success. Where would you put yourself on this spectrum of opinion?

All the delegates agreed that a well-developed sense of humour is essential!

Separating qualities from skills is not easy, but for convenience we might agree this distinction: skills can be learned but qualities are innate and can only be developed. Look again at the qualities you listed for yourself; try to determine which could be further developed.

Good quality care, in whatever sphere, needs a high degree of self-awareness on the part of carer or practitioner: if we are not aware of how we affect others, we are unlikely to improve our interactions with others. Clinical supervision provides an excellent forum for the development of self-awareness in both parties and thus also encourages development of qualities. Let's look in greater depth at some of the qualities advocated by butterworth and faugier in order to clarify the supervisor's role. As you read about each, evaluate how important the quality is and whether you could develop it in yourself.

Generous

Supervisors need to be generous in at least two ways. Firstly, supervisors need to be generous with their time. In palliative care work, as in other care work, or in teaching (perhaps in any profession) time is at a premium. It is in some senses the most precious commodity we have, with a special urgency in care of the dying and those nearest to them. It may be difficult for supervisors to allocate time for clinical supervision, especially if they see other tasks as having greater and higher priority. This can sometimes result in the supervisees feeling rather discouraged, because they wonder if they are being some sort of nuisance. Careful allocation of time for clinical supervision meetings is therefore an important aspect of the clinical supervision 'contract' and supervisors need to believe in the value and importance of this work and to allocate time accordingly. Research confirms that being generous with time for clinical supervision yields worthwhile rewards. Secondly, supervisors need what might be called 'generosity of spirit'. It can be very difficult (and not very rewarding) to be supervised by someone who is not prepared to 'give'. How would you describe a 'giving' person?

✐ **Your thoughts**

How would you describe a giving person?

Supervisors need to 'give' intellectually and emotionally. If clinical supervision is to inspire higher standards, the genuine *sharing* of knowledge, experience and expertise is crucial.

✐ **Your thoughts**

How important is it to be generous?
How could you develop this quality further in yourself?

Rewarding

An important supervisor skill, which we look at in detail in a later chapter, is the ability to give **feedback**. Feedback is different from praise, as we shall see, but the ability to give appropriate praise and encouragement is also a very helpful quality in a supervisor. Most of us work (and live) more comfortably if we feel approved of and have a sense that our contribution is valued. Here is what an experienced, mature oncology nurse said during her own clinical supervision:

👁 **Witness statement**

If I remember one thing from my early days, it's Sister —. Everyone felt good on her ward, and we were all willing to go that extra mile. She never went off duty, or let you go off, without saying 'Thank you' and giving some genuine word of appreciation.

It is interesting that this nurse (now a palliative care sister herself) uses the word 'genuine'. Praise that is formulaic will not help the working alliance and so will not contribute to the sense of well-being that raises standards.

✎ **Your thoughts**

How important is it to be rewarding?
How could you develop this quality further in yourself?

Thoughtful and thought-provoking

Clinical supervision is set-aside time that offers a valuable opportunity for reflecting on practice, but much of the opportunity will be wasted if the parties do not use it to share **thinking** about practice. This implies a measure of preparation. Supervisors need to challenge themselves intellectually. Clinical supervision is (in part) a learning forum, and in order to challenge supervisees, supervisors need to challenge themselves, and to reflect on their own practice, both as palliative care practitioners and as supervisors. A supervisor who is ready to learn, especially one who is willing and ready to learn from a supervisee, is likely to create a good learning environment. This willingness to learn also helps to dispel any anxieties about hierarchy.

Research seems to show that having good role models is one of the most powerful learning tools and one of the best ways of improving practice. A supervisor who is thinking about issues and about his or her own practice will inspire similar intellectual growth in a supervisee.

Humanity and sensitivity

Professions which involve care are, by their very nature, involved with the 'ups and downs' and joys and sorrows of other people in a variety of ways – nurses provide intimate physical care, and moreover workers in palliative care are privileged to accompany people on probably the most difficult journey they can make. You will be able to think of many more examples of this special involvement.

Patients and clients at these vulnerable times need to have their dignity respected, and a good supervisor will model this by the way in which patients and clients are discussed in the clinical supervision sessions. A supervisor who has this quality will also be sensitive to the supervisee's need for respect and dignity. If supervisees are to bring to clinical supervision not only their successes, but also what they see as their 'failures' (and the guilt that so often goes with these) they need to be confident that the supervisor will view their work with sensitivity. The clinical supervision session is not an appraisal, and much less is it a disciplinary session, so a real understanding that sometimes despite our best efforts things do go wrong calls for sensitive handling by the supervisor, if real learning is to result.

Uncompromising

This may be a difficult quality to develop. We said that clinical supervision is not an appraisal, much less some kind of disciplinary interview. (You may be interested to know that some managers have, mistakenly, used clinical supervision as some kind of threat. I have myself had supervisees say, resentfully or truculently, something like, 'I've been told I *have* to have clinical supervision.' Working through this is not an easy route to a working alliance!) Since the main purpose of clinical supervision is to improve and enhance patient and client care, then it follows that examination and discussion of standards will form part of the work. What does the word uncompromising mean for you?

🖉 Your thoughts

What does the term 'uncompromising' mean to you?

It is unfortunate that the word may have negative associations. People who are 'uncompromising' may be seen as being unprepared to accept any kind of change or even as being downright stubborn! This is not, you'll be glad to hear, the sense of 'uncompromising' that applies to the clinical supervisor! It has more to do with the sense that the supervisor can model a rigorous approach to standards. This can be a vital contribution to the process of clinical supervision – to raise standards from 'good enough' to 'good', from 'good' to 'very good' and then to 'excellent' demands an uncompromising approach to the standards required in palliative care. Some supervisors may find it difficult to sustain the warmth and trust that goes along with the humanity and sensitivity we discussed previously with this quality of being uncompromising about standards; much will depend on the supervisors ability to develop an atmosphere of trust, based on appropriate confidentiality.

Reflect on this witness statement, given by a palliative care nurse supervisee:

👁 Witness statement

There was one patient who, try as I might, I just couldn't 'take to'. And to be truthful I didn't care much for his relatives. The whole family were aggressive and unreasonably demanding. I told my supervisor about *what* I was doing which I was confident was of a high standard. Even so, she sensed that I was confused and concerned that somehow I wasn't doing enough, even though I'd just given her a lengthy description of what I *was* doing! She suggested that we look together at what palliative care means, especially the holistic aspect.

It soon dawned on me that it wasn't what I was doing, but how I was *doing* it which was lacking. I don't know to this day how she did it, but I do know that my attitude to the patient changed because, in a way, she had challenged my beliefs. She did sympathise with my inability to like the patient, but she didn't let the sympathy affect an uncompromising stance about standards.

Reviewing all of these qualities (and there are so many more that we could explore) highlights the fact that a supervisor has a dual responsibility:

- She or he is **responsible for** monitoring the standard of the Supervisee's work and how this affects patient or client care, but in rather a different way from a line manager. The supervisor is responsible for doing this through a relationship of trust, built on confidence, confidentiality and respect. As Hawkins and Shohet put it, supervisors 'keep open the space in which people can learn and grow' and are 'servants of the process' (Hawkins and Shohet, 1989)

- There is variation in whom supervisors are **responsible to**. They have a responsibility to managers or whoever is giving them time and space to carry out their supervision. They may also have a responsibility, if they are working independently, to whoever is paying them. In counselling (and most palliative care teams have a counsellor member) this may well be the supervisee himself or herself, which may add to the complexity of the role. And of course supervisors have a responsibility to whatever profession they represent to maintain standards and integrity.

Perhaps you could re-visit what you thought about responsibility in *Chapter One* and reflect on whether your views have changed at all.

The supervisee

In the literature about supervision and clinical supervision very little has been explored about the role and responsibilities of the supervisee. It is almost as if all the work will be done by the supervisor, and indeed that can sometimes be a danger. However, if clinical supervision is to be a genuine working *alliance* there must be at least two working partners. Similarly if clinical supervision is to be a learning forum, they will be teacher and learner – and in good clinical supervision these roles should be interchangeable, as each partner is learning from the other.

Take a moment to list the qualities you think should be present in supervisees if they are to gain from supervision.

✏ **Your thoughts**

What qualities do you think a supervisee should have?

Here are some of the qualities I would hope to find in myself as a supervisee and that I would be looking for in anyone I might be asked to supervise. I would like a supervisee to:

- understand what clinical supervision is (means)
- be willing to enter into the process
- be keen to learn
- be open to new ideas (especially about palliative care)
- be reflective about practice and committed to high standards in it
- be honest
- appreciate the fact that a need for support does not indicate weakness
- be self-aware (which perhaps sums up all the others).

How do our lists compare?

The first two qualities go hand in hand – if a potential supervisee has an unfortunate view of clinical supervision and sees it as the negative activity we mentioned in *Chapter One*, then it is unlikely that she or he will enter into the process. It seems important then that some kind of preliminary discussion to clarify terms and meaning should take place before the supervisee begins working with a supervisor (we examine this again in a later chapter). The supervisor might take responsibility for clarifying the nature of clinical supervision, but it will be up to the supervisee to understand the function and appreciate that they are entering into a working *alliance*.

Adults seem to learn in a very different way from children, and the mutual learning which should take place in clinical supervision may be very different from how we learned as children, or even from how we trained for our professional roles. Research indicates that adults learn best when they actively engage in the learning process and when they decide for themselves what they want to learn. The term 'self-managed learning' has been used to describe this type of learning, and perhaps we could term it 'taking responsibility'. Self-managing in the clinical supervision learning forum should lead to openness to new ideas and ways of being.

This comes from John Bowlby (1980), whose work is so important for understanding the losses associated with palliative care:

> *The painfulness of new ideas and our habitual resistance to them can be seen... The more far-reaching a new idea, the more disorganisation of existing theoretical systems has to be tolerated before a better synthesis of old and new can be achieved.*

A practitioner who is not open to considering new perspectives (even if they are, after some thought, rejected) is unlikely to make a reflective practitioner. If we never reflect on our practice, how do we know that it is good and that it is meeting the standards of our profession? How can we learn from anything that might go wrong? How can we develop? A supervisee who comes to clinical supervision with no desire to learn through reflection will not benefit from the working alliance.

The following anecdote links the two qualities we have just explored with yet another quality – honesty.

👁 **Witness statement**

In his own clinical supervision, a supervisor disclosed that he was finding it very difficult to work with his supervisee – a hospice palliative care nurse:
'Every time she comes she tells me all the wonderful things she's been doing, and some of them are indeed excellent and I don't stint my praise – but she NEVER brings anything else. I don't just mean failures, but never anything that she's read or heard about that might affect her practice. I have tried to challenge her and point her towards articles and so on that I've found interesting, but she just doesn't seem to 'hear' what I'm saying. Somehow I can see her being like this in ten years' time... I do wonder about her trust in me

---

A supervisee's responsibility is to bring to clinical supervision sessions an honest willingness to reflect on practice and to learn. As a prospective supervisee, ask yourself the following questions.

✎ **Your thoughts**

How do you know that your practice is more than 'good enough'?
How satisfied are you with your work? With the organisation you work for?
Are there any deficits in your skills? How will you make good any gaps?
Is there anything or anybody you find very hard to cope with?
If you could change one thing about your work, what would it be?
Where do you see yourself in ten years' time?

Being prepared to use supervision sessions to explore issues like these can fulfil the formative and perspective functions of clinical supervision, as well as being restorative, but although the supervisor can be a 'sounding board' or guide, he or she can only work with what the supervisee brings.

One of the questions you reflected on (is there anything you find very hard to cope with?) Raises a further point about supervisee qualities. Working with people, especially ill, troubled or stressed people – and even more so when working with the dying – is very tiring.

A curious myth seems to have arisen, whereby people who are not 'stressed out' are not really working as hard as they should. Conversely, people who seem to have got their work–life balance right often complain that they are seen as 'not pulling their weight' and can be regarded with a degree of suspicion as being lazy. It is quite difficult to see how this myth has developed, but it has led to a very unfortunate result – seeking help or support is somehow regarded as 'weak'. This was summed up thus by Dass (1995):

> *Many helpers when they themselves are suffering are incapable of accepting support or at least receiving it easily. Yet they may be impatient with those they are working with for not accepting aid or counselling readily enough. Chances are – if you cannot accept help, you cannot really give it.*

✎ **Your thoughts**

What do you think about this failure to accept help or support?

In *Chapter One* we quoted Ruskin's view that to be happy in our work we should not do too much of it. Taking time out to review our work and our work–life balance is not self-indulgent – it is an essential aspect of maintaining good health. The benefits of good work–life balance are well researched and we can be clear about the advantages for physical and mental well-being. The structured one-hour-a-month of clinical supervision is an appropriate and productive means of achieving this.

Pause for a moment and jot down your thoughts about the following points.

✐ Your thoughts

In your work environment is there a sort of hidden culture that if you aren't exhausted, then you can't be working hard enough?

What is the attitude towards people who are assertive and say 'No' when asked repeatedly to do more than their fair share of work? (notice that the question asks 'repeatedly')

How often do people stagger in to work when they're really not fit enough? Are they seen as saints or heroes?

What are your own beliefs and values about seeking support? For others? For yourself?

The supervisee qualities, just as those of the supervisor, could be summed up as **self-awareness**. Very few of us know ourselves, and in our work, if we are to avoid upsetting others, or perhaps labelling them because of our own values and beliefs, biases and prejudices, we need to be as self-aware as possible. Clinical supervision offers an environment where we can safely explore our attitudes and value systems and gain some insight into how these might appear to others and how they might be affected by them.

✐ Your thoughts

What do you understand by the term 'therapeutic use of self' which has become quite common in care and palliative care 'language'?

In palliative care, in nursing in general, in other care work, and perhaps in any work that involves interaction with others, the most powerful tool that we have is ourselves. The way we *are* with others, whether they are patients, clients, students, colleagues, is fundamental to the help that we can give them. Clinical supervision can help us to examine how we operate interpersonally, so that we become aware of our 'blind spots', grow in self-awareness and so use ourselves more therapeutically.

Just for fun, work through the following 'driver' questionnaire to see how well you know yourself.

☞ 'Driver' questionnaire

This is not a personality test. It is intended to stimulate your awareness of the ways you cause yourself stress. Answer 'Yes', 'No' or 'To some extent' and then score 1 for 'Yes', ½ for 'To some extent' and 0 for 'No'.

1. Do you set yourself high standards, and then criticise yourself for failing to meet them?
2. Is it important to you to be RIGHT?
3. Do you feel irritated or annoyed by small messes, or things out of place?
4. Do you hate to be interrupted?
5. Do you like to explain things in detail and precisely?

6. Do you do things for others that you don't really want to do?
7. Is it important for you to be LIKED?
8. Are you fairly easily persuaded?
9. Do you dislike being different?
10. Do you dislike conflict?

11. Do you have a tendency to do a lot of things simultaneously?
12. Would you describe yourself as 'quick' and find yourself getting impatient with others?
13. Do you tend to talk at the same time as others, or finish their sentences for them?
14. Do you like to 'get on with the job' rather than talk about it?
15. Do you set unrealistic time limits? (especially ones that are too short?)

16. Do you hide or control your feelings?
17. Are you reluctant to ask for help?
18. Do you have a tendency to put yourself (or find yourself) in the position of being depended upon?

---

19. Do you have a tendency not to realise how hungry, tired or ill you are, but instead 'keep going'?
20. Do you prefer to do things on your own?

21. Do you hate 'giving up' or 'giving in', always hoping this time it will work?
22. Do you have a tendency to start things and not finish them?
23. Do you tend to compare yourself (or your performance) with others, and feel inferior or superior accordingly?
24. Do you find yourself going round in circles with a problem, feeling stuck but unable to let go of it?
25. Do you have a tendency to be 'the rebel' or the 'odd one out' in a group?

A further way of assessing self-awareness is to use the Johari window. You will find a diagram of this in the addendum at the end of the chapter, and a full explanation can be found in *Counselling Skills for Palliative Care* (Bayliss 2004).

In a very real sense then the supervisee is responsible for bringing him or her *self* to the supervision sessions.

Supervisees, just like supervisors, have a complex range of responsibilities. They are responsible to and for their patients and clients and for the work that they do with and for them. They are responsible to their employing organisation (or the voluntary organisation which they represent). They are responsible to their professional organisations, and for the code(s) of ethics and practice set by them.

You can see that the roles and responsibilities of both supervisors and supervisees mean that clinical supervision is much more than a bit of a chat each month!

As a final exercise in this chapter imagine yourself first as a supervisee and then as a supervisor.

✐ Your thoughts

As a supervisee what would you look for in a supervisor? And what would you bring to supervision?
As a supervisor what would you expect from a supervisee? And what could you offer in clinical supervision?

References

Bayliss J (2004) *Counselling Skills in Palliative Care*. Quay Books, London

Bowlby J (1980) *Attachment and Loss*. Basic Books, New York

Butterworth T, Faugier J (1992) *Clinical Supervision and Mentoring in Nursing*, 1st edn. Chapman and Hall, London

Dass (1995) *Compassion in Action: Setting Out on the Path of Service*, 2nd edn. Three Rivers Press, Michigan

Hawkins P, Shohet R (1989) *Supervision in the Helping Professions*. Open University Press, Milton Keynes

Addendum to Chapter Two

The Johari window

	KNOWN TO SELF		UNKNOWN TO SELF
KNOWN TO OTHERS	'Open'	Feed-back	'Blind'
	Self-disclosure	INSIGHT	
UNKNOWN TO OTHERS	'Hidden'		'Unknown'

1. 'Open' area – to self and others, 'on top of table'
2. 'Blind' area – unknown to self but apparent to others
3. 'Hidden' area – known to self, hidden to others, 'under the table'
4. 'Unknown' area – to self and to others, potential available but not yet discovered

CHAPTER 3

Re-visiting functions and exploring models

An NHS primary care trust was in the process of implementing clinical supervision. Here is a statement made by a senior nurse at one of the preliminary meetings that had been organised to familiarise staff with the concept:

👁 Witness statement

But what is it *for*? It's not that I don't agree with it, but I don't see what clinical supervision can do that we don't do now. I can always have a chat with my staff; they know that they can come to me – my door is always open so to speak – and there's a proper process for dealing with complaints if anything goes wrong. So what is clinical supervision actually *for*?

Look back at the elements of clinical supervision that we explored in *Chapter One*:

- Formative
- Normative
- Restorative
- Perspective

✐ Your thoughts

How might you have answered this nurse and helped to calm her anxieties?

It is interesting that the findings of a two-year research programme into clinical supervision recorded that seventy per cent of all participants who were receiving clinical supervision were 'overwhelmingly positive about the experience'. The research highlighted several benefits experienced by the research participants; one of the most striking was a significant increase in job satisfaction.

Job satisfaction

☞ Minnesota Job Satisfaction Scale

According to Butterworth *et al* (1997) results from the Minnesota Job Satisfaction Scale show that:

- There was a decreased satisfaction score until clinical supervision was introduced in the second time band of the research and the satisfaction score stabilised in the third time band.
- When clinical supervision was removed from one group after the second time band, job satisfaction decreased significantly in the third time band.
- Participants who received clinical supervision throughout the research had a higher satisfaction score by the third time band.

Job satisfaction is clearly of benefit to a supervisee. We spend a great deal of our time and expend much energy – both physical and emotional – on work. This expenditure of time and energy is made worthwhile by the degree of satisfaction which the work provides. Working in palliative care provides unique possibilities and opportunities for job satisfaction, although some people find it difficult to understand how palliative care workers can derive satisfaction and even fulfilment from working with the dying and those closest to them. The box below lists some comments that I have heard or which have been addressed to me.

◉ Witness statements

How can you bear seeing people die all the time?
Doesn't it get you down – all that sadness?
I couldn't do your job – I went into nursing to help people get better.
What do you do to get away from it?

Try to list what satisfactions you derive from working in palliative care.

✐ **Your thoughts**

Which elements of palliative care will give you job satisfaction?

Clinical supervision, as the research shows us, can enhance job satisfaction, especially perhaps in its restorative function. Job satisfaction is closely linked to sickness rates. The information below describes some recent health commission findings on sickness and absenteeism among hospital-based nurses. Record your personal views as to why sickness rates seem so high for nurses.

✐ **Your thoughts**

Healthcare Commission concerns over absenteeism in nurses

The Healthcare Commission conducted a survey of 135 000 hospital ward staff, including registered nurses, nursing auxiliaries and healthcare assistants, in 6000 British hospitals. They calculated that ward nurses took more days of sick then most other public sector staff, at a cost approaching £500 million each year!

In their survey, ward staff members took an average of 16.8 days off work per year, with unqualified ward staff taking much more, an average of 21.4 days sick leave each year. In the public sector the average yearly figure was much lower, at just 11.3 days. This means that ward nurses took more days off than most other groups, including social workers (16.1 days), prison officers (14.7 days), council workers (10.7 days), police officers (10.4 days), civil servants (10 days), and teachers (just 5.4 days).

According to the Commission, these sickness levels are 'unacceptably high'. Blame has been placed on various factors including stress, low job satisfaction, pressures caused by NHS reforms, and the heavy workload and the physical nature of the job, which lead to several occupational disorders ranging from low back pain to back strain and needlestick injury.

cont../.

The precise causes for these high rates of absenteeism remain unclear, but it seems hospitals are employing more and more temporary and agency staff, both to fill vacancies and to cover for sickness and holiday leave. The Commission predicts savings of nearly £150 million a year if the sickness rate could be reduced by thirty per cent.

What are your views about absenteeism among nurses?

Clearly sickness and absence have serious financial implications, not only for the NHS, but for hospices and for other charities providing palliative care. The graph (*Figure 3.1*) Shows the effects of clinical supervision on sickness rates.

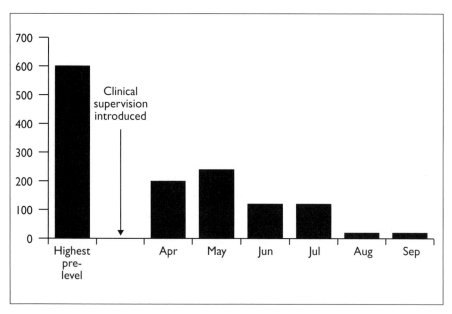

Figure 3.1: Staff sickness hours – pre-clinical and post-clinical supervision

The research which produced this information, and which included palliative care workers, seems to show conclusively that clinical supervision can have a significant effect on absence rates. The economic benefits of this for employers, managers, and organisers are evident. More importantly, there is likely to be a significant effect on patient care. Patients, and the people closest to them, seem to value *consistent* care. It is as if they become attached to their carers and find changes caused by absence stressful and, sometimes, distressing. Occasionally this dislike of change can show itself as resentment; we may see this as irrational but it is very real for some of the people we aim to help.

Look at the following two statements given specifically for this chapter.

👁 Witness statements

The husband of a patient receiving hospice-at-home palliative care
It was difficult really. It took ages for my wife to get used to the one nurse doing all those intimate things for her. Then she went off with back trouble and for a little while we had a succession of different people. Don't get me wrong – they were all very good, but we didn't know from one day to the next who might turn up, even though we were very grateful to whoever came. I could see the effect on my wife, and to tell the truth, it affected me, too – I just couldn't seem to open up in the same way that I had with _____. I'd got to trust her, you see.

A 'bank' nurse working with palliative care patients in their homes, in clinical supervision:
When you take over from someone on a temporary basis, it can be very difficult. not always, of course. In a way it's a tribute to the permanent person that the patients miss her or him, but a few seem to think it's my fault that they're on leave or off sick, and then it's really difficult to build up rapport. And of course you yourself may not be around for very long. I don't know what the answer is, but it's not easy to feel that you're some sort of intruder and that they'd prefer their usual person.

Since clinical supervision can have such a major impact on sickness or absence rates, it would appear that it can have an organisational function, as well as the four 'individual' functions we have already reviewed. Therefore, this has a strong 'knock-on' effect to quality of care, as the two witness statements highlight.

Clinical governance

Palliative care providers, particularly if they are hospital-based, are subject to both professional and political 'drivers'. Clinical governance has perhaps been the most encompassing of these. The Department of Health (DoH, 1998a,b) defined clinical governance as:

> *... a framework through which NHS organisations are responsible for continuously improving the quality of their services and safeguarding high standards of care by creating an environment in which excellence in clinical care will flourish.*

and:

> *... the means by which organisations ensure the provision of quality clinical care by making individuals accountable for setting, maintaining and monitoring performance standards.*

Clinical governance thus places the responsibility for quality of care on organisations *and* on individuals within those organisations. *Organisations* are responsible for ensuring that the services they provide are of a high standard and this has to be demonstrated by setting standards which ensure that individual clinicians fulfil their individual responsibilities. They should also monitor the systems they have set up.

Individuals (clinicians and other palliative care workers/practitioners) are responsible for providing high quality care and must be able to *demonstrate* this.

The level of accountability for both organisations and individuals is high. Take a moment to consider whether in your palliative care setting there is (as was the intention of clinical governance) a formal link between the organisation and the individual practitioner, particularly in your own setting.

✐ Your thoughts

In your palliative care setting, is there a formal link between the organisation and the individual practitioner?

Look back at the definitions of clinical supervision that we listed in *Chapter One*. The Department of Health's definition (DoH, 1998a,b) is:

> *... a formal process of professional support and learning which enables individual practitioners to develop knowledge and competence, assume responsibility for their own practice and enhance consumer protection and safety of care in complex clinical situations.*

Whilst this acknowledges the (increasing) complexity of care and emphasises the need for accountability, it does not suggest how these might be linked to clinical governance. There is an increasing body of opinion which believes that the crucial link is provided by clinical supervision. Where clinical supervision exists or is being established, there is clear evidence that matters brought to supervision sessions by supervisees focus strongly on issues of crucial importance to an organisation. Providing clinical supervision is therefore a clear demonstration that an organisation is effective in clinical governance, while participation in clinical supervision demonstrates the desired individual responsibility.

Team work

There are many examples of how the two can be linked. Work through the following chart of 'drivers' and in the fourth column comment on how the initiatives might help in your own palliative care setting (*Table 3.1*).

Pause for a moment and look again at the more light-hearted 'Driver' questionnaire you completed in *Chapter Two*.

Think about your palliative care colleagues and how you might answer those questions for each member of your team.

Palliative care is, arguably, the care provision which is most reliant on team work. Take a minute to list what you see as the characteristics of a good, effective palliative care team:

✐ **Your thoughts**

What are the characteristics of a good and effective palliative care team?

Table 3.1: The key professional and political drivers and their link to Clinical Supervision

Professional and political drivers	Aims of organisation	Relevance to clinical supervision	How might this initiative help in your setting?
UKCC, United Kingdom Central Council for Nursing, Midwifery and Health Visiting (now the Nursing and Midwifery Council, NMC)	Professional body that protects public from unsafe practice	The Code of Practice and standards set out by the UKCC/NMC must be adhered to at all times both within and outside clinical supervision sessions	
PREP, post-registration education and practice	All qualified nurses are required to demonstrate they have received at least five days education in every three-year period of registration. Not all learning will be undertaken in a formal setting	Identifies and addresses improvements in any individual's performance	
Our Healthier Nation (Department of Health, 1998)	Focuses on clear targets for improving health of the nation. Specific target areas are: • Heart disease and stroke • Reducing accidents • Cancer • Mental health	Key targets can be used as a focus for clinical supervision sessions	
White Paper: The new NHS modern dependable (Department of Health, 1997)	Sets out Government strategy for how the health service will be managed. Focuses on collaboration and partnership, to deliver high quality, cost-effective health care	Clinical supervision provides an arena to discuss the impact of the document and supports health care professionals in implementing the changes	

Table 3.1 continued

Professional and political drivers	Aims of organisation	Relevance to clinical supervision	How might this initiative help in you setting?
A First Class Service: Quality in the new NHS (Department of Health, 1998a)	Focuses on the quality agenda. Main themes include: • Clinical governance • National service frameworks • National Institute for Clinical Excellence • Evidence-based practice • Continued professional development • Professional self-regulation	Of all the most recent documents, this will have most impact on the professional at practice level. Clinical governance will be one of the main drivers for clinical supervision as participation demonstrates individuals exercising their responsibility, which is a key feature of this framework	
Working Together, Securing a Quality Workforce for the NHS (Department of Health, 1998b)	Aims to ensure that NHS employees are able to make the best possible contribution to improving health and patient care. Focuses on: • Fairness • Equality • Flexibility • Leadership skills • Life-long learning • Recruitment and retention	Clinical supervision will allow exploration of these issues and development of partnerships both from within the organisation and outside. Clinical supervision can assist in ensuring that staff are valued and supported, thus promoting a healthy workforce	

In our working (and private) lives we will have belonged to many teams of one sort or another, and some will have been more effective than others. The qualities which make for an effective team seem to obtain for most work, and are especially relevant to palliative care, because of the essential aspect of holistic care which we aim to provide. Good teams are effective in several ways: they carry out their tasks efficiently and well; the members work well together and a purposeful atmosphere seems to prevail; the individual members seem to gain personal satisfaction from belonging to the team.

Here is how a team of Macmillan nurses described the characteristics of their team:

- good atmosphere within the team
- good communication
- the team is clear about what it is doing
- an equal commitment from all team members
- the calibre of the team leader
- the way the team takes decisions.

No doubt you can add to the list from your own experience. Of course different teams will have their individual strengths and weaknesses.

In a *Team Development Manual* (Woodcock, 1989) nine 'building blocks' are suggested as vital for team effectiveness. Effective teams:

- are clear about what they want to achieve
- confront issues and resolve them in an open way
- have an atmosphere of support and trust
- can use both co-operation and conflict to get results
- have clear procedures for taking decisions
- are led in a way that suits the task, the team and individual members
- regularly review what they are doing and learn from this
- encourage individuals to develop
- relate well to other teams.

Keeping patient focus in a group with the many different approaches which can be present in a palliative care team (nurses, managers, counsellors, volunteers, social workers, and doctors, for example) is not easy. It is probably inevitable that from time to time conflict will arise. The ability to contain and to use positively any conflict can be greatly helped by clinical supervision, whether it is conducted individually or in a group.

Look at the following chart, which was used in group clinical supervision to help a hospice team which did not feel that it was functioning as effectively as it could (or should). You might like to fill it in for the team to which you belong.

☞ Team assessment of value of clinical supervision

Members were asked to give a score of 1 to 6 (6 is very good indeed) for their team against the listed criteria.

- Is the team clear about what it wants to achieve
  (short and long term)? ☐
- Does the team confront issues and deal with them openly? ☐
- Do members of the team support and trust each other? ☐
- Is the team able to use both co-operation and conflict to
  achieve results? ☐
- Does the team have a procedure for reaching consensus/decisions? ☐
- Is the team led in a way that suits the task, the team, and
  individuals? ☐
- Does the team review what it does on a regular basis? ☐
- Are individual able to develop within the team? ☐
- Does the team relate well with other teams? ☐

After scoring members were asked to write a few sentences about how they would like clinical supervision to help the issues which the scores had revealed.

It was only in the confidential forum of clinical supervision that team members felt able to discuss problems openly. The happy outcome was a much more effective team and, of course, an effective team leads to improved patient care. We have noted that sick leave can have financial implications, which may often have a 'knock on' effect for patient care. Financial concerns may also be a cause of some conflict in teams. Palliative care in the UK and in hospices especially, is highly dependent upon charitable giving. You may be able to cite many fund raising efforts locally to you aimed at supporting palliative care, and are perhaps engaged in some yourself. One nurse manager of a day hospice expressed her thoughts to me as shown in the box below.

👁 Witness statement

When all is said and done, this place runs on jumble sales.

Anxiety about resources and about resource management can create conflict in teams as members will each have their own priorities and even their own ideologies as to what is 'good' for a dying person or what is in his or her 'best interest'.

Read the following case study which illustrates how resource constraints can create conflict. It is part of an audiotape transcription of a team discussion at a hospice and it is used with their consent. After some specific patient/case discussion the weekly meeting moved on to more general issues. The education/training officer wanted to expand the library and to take over a room currently used for activities – painting, craftwork, meditation and some complementary therapies – for study and tutorial work.

👁 Witness statements

Education officer In the long term, it will be better use, because the more people we train and educate the more help we'll get, and that's bound to benefit patients.

Volunteer co-ordinator Yes, I see your point, but what about *now*? The patients, I mean the ones we've got, really benefit from the activities. What's supposed to happen to them? And there's the volunteers ...

Nurse Yes, and I wonder who reads all these books anyway – most of us don't have time.

Administrator It's true, though, that training days do bring in quite a bit of money, and if we could have more study days or run more courses then ...

Education officer That's my point exactly!

Other nurse But are we supposed to be *educating* people? I thought we were here to support dying people and their families. That's why I'm here anyway.

Education officer Yes, but ...

Administrator The building only has so many rooms and we only have so much money – It's a tightrope.

The meeting became quite heated and ended with no clear outcome or resolution and with quite a few hurt feelings. Really good clinical supervision (had this been group supervision) would have attempted to *use* this conflict – after all, it generated a great deal of energy, and that energy could have been used creatively. Jot down what you think a skilled supervisor might have offered here, as opposed to what a chairperson might have done (although this team did not have a chairperson, but there was an obvious leader).

✎ **Your thoughts**

What might a skilled supervisor have offered in this situation?

As well as ensuring 'equal air time' for team members, a supervisor would have worked to explore *shared* responsibilities (it is clear from the extract that members were each following a personal agenda). He or she would also have needed to confront inconsistencies and to ensure that any consensus was accepted and, if not, that members were aware of the implications. At the same time their own views would need to be kept hidden for fear of bias, although offering experience gained elsewhere might have been helpful. Very often, teams seem to find themselves in an 'either/or' situation:

either
We promote education
or
We provide complementary activities

when often both can be achieved. The clinical supervision function of **perspective** is crucial here, and clearly the role it can play in promoting more effective team work (and hence better care) is important.

Clinical supervision, then, has an organisational function as well as a personal one. There is some evidence that it helps with recruitment and retention, too, which is obviously an advantage in both spheres. Another benefit for organisations is that complaints seem to decrease where there is effective clinical supervision. This has a dramatic effect on morale, and the general benefit of high morale is obvious. In practical terms too there is a benefit – investigating complaints is costly and time consuming and can be very damaging to team spirit and ethos, so the fewer complaints there are the more the service will benefit.

Models of supervision

The success of clinical supervision may depend to a large extent on the model which is used. When clinical supervision is introduced or implemented, it makes very sound sense to consult about which model is preferred.

The box below gives several examples of the ways in which clinical supervision may be conducted. As you examine each, try to think of the advantages and disadvantages for yourself a) as a supervisee, b) as a supervisor c) as a team member.

☞ **MODEL 1. Regular one-to-one sessions with supervisor from you own discipline**
a) As a supervisee
b) As a supervisor
c) As a team member
Advantages:
Disadvantages:

MODEL 2. Regular one-to-one sessions with supervisor from a different discipline
a) As a supervisee
b) As a supervisor
c) As a team member
Advantages:
Disadvantages:

MODEL 3. One-to-one peer supervision
a) As a supervisee
b) As a supervisor
c) As a team member
Advantages:
Disadvantages:

MODEL 4. Group supervision within your own discipline
a) As a supervisee
b) As a supervisor
c) As a team member
Advantages:
Disadvantages:

MODEL 5. Group supervision in a hybrid group
a) As a supervisee
b) As a supervisor
c) As a team member
Advantages:
Disadvantages:

MODEL 6. Peer-group supervision
a) As a supervisee
b) As a supervisor
c) As a team member
Advantages:
Disadvantages:

MODEL 7. Network supervision*
a) As a supervisee
b) As a supervisor
c) As a team member
Advantages:
Disadvantages:

MODEL 8. Triad supervision*
a) As a supervisee
b) As a supervisor
c) As a team member
Advantages:
Disadvantages:

* For an explanation of these models see text body.

The models are mostly self-explanatory, but a word of explanation about the last two terms, network supervision and triad supervision, may be helpful.

Network supervision involves linking up with others involved in the same kind of work (in our case palliative care), but not from the same organisation. For example, two or three hospices, or maybe bereavement care helpers in an area might link up. An obvious disadvantage could be the complications that arise simply in organisation of the meetings; an obvious advantage might be the generation of fresh ways of looking at work from others' perspectives. Confidentiality might also be an issue. One enthusiastic group I encountered while researching this book were using the internet and were considering videoconferencing.

Triad supervision involves (as its name implies) three people working together in each session. Each person takes an agreed role – supervisor, supervisee, and observer. All three members of the trio take a turn in each role, for an agreed length of time. In this way, feedback is received not only as a supervisee, but also on one's skill as a supervisor (given by the observer).

The box below shows some comments made by people who have experienced these different models. Their comments about the advantages and disadvantages may resonate with yours.

👁 **Witness statements**

Model 1. It was very helpful that my supervisor worked in the same field, because she, so to speak, used the same language, so I didn't have to explain anything and that speeded things up.

Model 2. At first I thought that having someone from a different discipline wouldn't work, but it is actually very good because it means I really have to explain my practice and when she asks me why I've done this or that I really reflect on my reasons. It's as if in explaining it to her, I explain it to myself.

Model 3. It was supposed to be clinical supervision, but it was more like case discussion – which we're having anyway. Maybe the problem was that neither of us had any training in how to do it.

Model 4. Group supervision is like our case meetings, but it's different, partly because our manager isn't there. Now that we trust each other we can really open up about our practice. It's taken quite a while though and the supervisor had to be very strong – especially about the contract which none of us thought was necessary to start with, but I can see now how important it was to have one.

Model 5. I like hearing other people's views about my patients. It's usually quite helpful, though our supervisor sometimes has a hard job keeping us on task and not letting us get too anecdotal!

Model 6. If you're not careful it can turn into a bit of a gossip shop, which would really be a waste of time. I used to get the feeling that we were not going anywhere. It was much better once we agreed that each time we met, someone would lead or would bring a paper to discuss.

Model 7. I'd love to try this. We only see staff from St _____'s once or twice a year. The trouble is we'd need a secretary or something to organise it and I don't see that happening!

Model 8. I've learned a lot – especially that I'm no good as an observer! I can do the other two roles (so I'm told) but I'm not good at giving feedback – still, I suppose that in itself is useful learning for my practice!

The eight models covered here could perhaps be described as practical models (we will look at models that are more process-based in a later chapter) and it is important to check out which suits each individual best. Shy or nervous people may find even small-group clinical supervision difficult or daunting and their valuable ideas about practice could get lost if the supervisor is not skilled. Issues of confidentiality can create difficulties in groups because they are so much more complex. Success will also depend upon the preferences (and availability) of the supervisor.

As a final exercise, look again at the senior nurse's statement at the front of the chapter. Consider how you might answer her now. Compare your thoughts with your original response. Is there a difference? If so, why do you think this is?

References

Bayliss VJ (2001) In: *Counselling Skills in Context*, Aldridge S, Rigby S (eds). Hodder and Stoughton, London

Butterworth T, Carson J, White E, Jeacock J, Clements A, Bishop V (1997) *It Is Good To Talk: An Evaluation Study of Clinical Supervision in England and Scotland*. University of Manchester, Manchester

Department of Health (1993) *A Vision for the Future. Report of the Chief Nursing Officer*. NHSME, London

Department of Health (1997) *White Paper: The new NHS modern dependable*. NHSE, London

Department of Health (1998a) *A First Class Service: Quality in the new NHS*. Health Service Circular 1998/113. NHSE, London

Department of Health (1998b) *Clinical Governance in North Thames. A paper for discussion and consultation*. NHSE North Thames Region Office, London

Department of Health (1998c) *Working Together, Securing a Quality Workforce for the NHS*. NHS executive

Woodcock M (1989) *Team Development Manual*. Gower, Hampshire

CHAPTER 4

The supervisor – qualities into skills

We begin this chapter (and could begin *Chapter Five* too) with a consideration of the nature of the supervisory relationship, which has been described as a 'microcosm of the wider society' (Butterworth and Faugier, 1994). What this description seems to imply is that the supervisory relationship is a sort of medium, through which a practitioner can analyse and reflect on many other relationships involved in their work.

Reflect for a moment on how many relationships you have as a palliative care worker.

✐ Your thoughts

How many relationships do you have with:

Patients and clients?
Colleagues? (list how many and how they are different)
Other relevant people?

Factors impacting on the supervisory relationship

The busy-ness of day-to-day work means that we often don't have time to analyse our interactions and relationships and to learn from them.

All relationships involve, to a greater or lesser degree, some kind of power issue, so being aware of this can have a profound effect on the supervisory relationship. There should be a very clear distinction between line management (what we might call managerial supervision) and clinical supervision (which may sometimes be called consultative supervision, but is still different). As we have said throughout, practitioners are unlikely to disclose mistakes, negative feelings about patients or colleagues, or fears and anxieties to someone who will have a powerful say in their next appraisal or be influential in their promotion prospects. The supervisory relationship should be non-hierarchical as this will ensure that the supervisor will learn from the supervisee, as well as the more obvious dynamic of the supervisee learning from the supervisor.

The power issue also needs to be considered in the way clinical supervision is implemented. The process may be introduced 'top down', which can lead to feelings of suspicion and even resentment; but 'bottom up' implementation can also present problems if practitioners consider themselves too busy to devise a coherent system. The impact of either on the supervisory relationship is likely to be negative. Look at what this ward manager of an oncology ward said to me:

◉ Witness statement

I do, actually, believe in clinical supervision, but I was just told to get it up and running by the autumn with no extra time to train people; no money to employ an external supervisor to kick us off. It wasn't surprising that there was no enthusiasm, to say the least!

Low enthusiasm is hardly a good omen for the supervisory relationship!

There are other factors which could impact on the supervisory relationship – these might be to do with gender, race, or culture. An antidiscriminatory way of working is inherent in palliative care, but there is a dearth of research into how antidiscriminatory practice operates in clinical supervision. One of the few studies (Cook and Helms, 1998) involved 225 supervisees from different ethnic backgrounds; all of them felt that (irrespective of the ethnic or cultural background of either supervisor or supervisee) feeling liked by the supervisor was the most important indicator of satisfaction with the process. Creating an atmosphere where the supervisee feels approved of and respected is obviously crucial to the success of the working alliance. The building of trust will be based on mutual respect, and although liking is not necessarily essential for respect, it certainly helps. Trust itself will depend on the nature and degree of confidentiality which exists within the relationship and we shall look at that in greater detail later, but both parties need to be clear about their boundaries *before* agreeing to work together. For example, it is not too difficult to know that confidentiality could and should be broken if malpractice is disclosed, but being clear about what is 'not good enough' practice is not so easily defined. Confusion about this sort of issue can have a very negative effect on the supervisory relationship.

Supervisors, as we shall see, need skills of contract making, but with so many factors affecting the relationship, it is often recommended that an exploratory meeting should take place, and only after that should both parties make a decision that they can and will work together. Here are some areas that might be covered in an exploratory discussion (you might like to add points that you would want to cover):

- The nature of the supervisee's entitlement and the terms of the service on offer, and how these match up.
- The supervisee's expectations of clinical supervision. If necessary clarify, modify or confirm these.
- Identification and exploration of any anxieties about clinical supervision (and these should be acknowledged and respected).
- Both parties' expectations about commitment.
- Clarification of ways of working.
- Exploration of the purpose and nature of working together (and agreement).
- Personal agenda

In *Chapter Two* we looked at the desirable *qualities* of a supervisor. Such qualities are essential but will not further the working alliance between the supervisor and supervisee unless they are communicated via a range of supervisory *skills*. As we have seen, some of these skills are needed preparatory to establishing the working alliance in order to clarify what the purpose of clinical supervision is. This is particularly necessary if the supervisee is hesitant about (or even hostile to!) The process. As some of the respondents in one of the first pieces of research into clinical supervision put it:

◉ Witness statement

The down side [of clinical supervision] is if it's not done in the spirit it should be carried out in. It will risk people feeling that there is a Big Brother. But I think that people are not used to being...I don't know...pro-actively managed. You see what I mean? They may find that if the relationship isn't right, that it is an intrusion and feel threatened by it. I think that it will need very careful handling.

cont../.

I tried to move people away from thinking it was a sort of punishment exercise, that it could be seen to guide, support, educate and develop staff. I would say that two of them perhaps are getting to the end of their careers, who would be referred to as 'old-style nurse managers', who have got very clear views – and have difficulty in seeing it as not punitive.

It's very difficult at the beginning to understand, you know, to go through it. You think 'Oh goodness, am I going to be watched all the time?' Because, I mean, supervision means 'supervise' doesn't it.

The biggest debate, probably, that we had was the term 'clinical supervision' and the fact that nobody within the group liked the word 'supervision'. Nobody likes it. Nobody could come up with a good alternative, but it was a major issue. I think that needs to be addressed at some point.

I can tell you that the name 'clinical supervision' is a stupid name. It's caused so many problems, I can't begin to tell you. Because people don't want to be thought of as being supervised – they feel you are looking, spying on them, you're trying to see what they are doing wrong, you are checking up on them, you're not in the capacity of an interested professional trying to support them and enhance their quality, skills and professional knowledge.

Counteracting such negativity will not be easy and it highlights how important that exploratory meeting is. So how might you have responded to some of these statements?

✐ Your thoughts

What would your response be to these negative statements?

On a more positive note, there have been reports of people at interview actually asking for assurances that they will be given clinical supervision, and opting for alternative posts if none is on offer. Given the recruitment problems in some areas of health care, this development is significant.

If there is an agreement to work together, some kind of contract needs to be agreed. The word 'contract' may sound rather formal but it is important to have an agreement and it is probably worth writing down what you have agreed to. Here is a list of what *might* be included. Think about each item and consider the implications for your own practice as a supervisor, or potential supervisor – what might you add, or take away?

Practical issues
- Time (length and frequency of sessions)
- Place
- Any costs involved and how these might affect the work
- Record taking and record keeping

Boundary issues
- Confidentiality (professional, patient/client, personal)
- Organisational limits/regulations
- Own contractual limitations (as a supervisor)
- Own level of competence

Ethical issues
- Codes of practice
- Access to records

Other issues
- Arrangements for giving feedback (to each other)
- Arrangements for reviewing how the clinical supervision work is progressing

---

✐ Your thoughts

What amendments, additions and deletions would you make as supervisor?

- To practical issues?
- To boundary issues?
- To ethical issues?
- To other issues?

The supervisee's responsibility

Practical issues

Although some of these items may seem obvious, even the simplest has implications. 'Time' for instance; this needs to be carefully considered – meeting when both parties are tired is less likely to be productive. Time may be especially problematic if group supervision is the chosen model, and this in turn affects supervisee commitment and responsibility. 'Place' can have serious implications for confidentiality, not only for the confidentiality between the supervisor and supervisee, but also for maintaining the confidentiality of patients or clients. 'Record taking' and 'record keeping' will certainly need clarifying, and we explore this in depth in a later chapter, as it is such a crucial and potentially difficult area.

If managers allocate time for clinical supervision, or perhaps fund an external supervisor, it is likely and indeed fair that they will require some sort of assurance that meetings are actually taking place. Some managers may be concerned to evaluate clinical supervision and to feel reassured that it is having a discernible effect on patient care or on some of the organisational issues we have considered. These concerns may affect the form and content of notes or records, so it is essential, as part of a contract, to agree on the format of notes and where they are to be kept.

Boundary issues

Boundary issues are likely to need a high level of clarification. Look at the following list of possibilities and try to reflect on how they might affect your personal practice as a clinical supervisor:

- The types of issues that are inappropriate for clinical supervision.
- The supervisee's views about what is or is not appropriate.
- The boundary between clinical supervision's restorative function and personal counselling.
- The limits of what can be provided (eg in terms of time or availability).
- The limits of one's own competence.
- The lines of accountability.
- The conflicts of responsibility and what to do about these.
- The conflicts of role.
- Confidentiality (of all parties involved).

✎ Your thoughts

How will your personal practice as a clinical supervisor be affected by these issues?

It is worth adding a word about that final point confidentiality – confidentiality should be *mutual*. Counsellors (and there is usually at least one counsellor on a palliative care team) are very accustomed to situations whereby, having carefully stated their own commitment to confidentiality, they find the client saying something like: 'I told my mother what you said, and she said...'.

In clinical supervision, there needs to be an agreement that both parties respect each other's confidentiality. This is so very important when the work is carried out within the relatively small sphere of palliative care, where other people may find it easy to identify who is being referred to, compared to the wider and more diverse world of care providers. Clarifying the limits of confidentiality is also an indicator of how open the clinical supervision will be: it would not be honest or fair to ignore those limits and later have to disclose them when trust had been established on a false basis.

Ethical issues

Ethical issues would certainly cover the codes of ethics and practice to which the parties adhere. In a palliative care team, nurses would be bound by the UKCC's code (now the NMC), and counsellors would probably adhere to the BACP's *Ethical Framework for Good Practice in Counselling and Psychotherapy* (BACP, 2001). The codes of both stipulate the limits to confidentiality, as well as giving guidance on ethical practice.

Try to read (or re-read) these codes and reflect on how the guidance about confidentiality might affect your practice as a supervisor. Codes of practice are closely linked to the normative function of clinical supervision, and you might find it helpful to re-visit the codes with this function in mind.

✎ Your thoughts

How does the code's guidance on confidentiality affect your practice as a supervisor?

Other members of a palliative care team may adhere to other and different codes. Clarifying these, and discussing the implications for the clinical supervision process is best considered as part of the contract, because it will ensure that any possible areas of conflict are sorted out and can be avoided later on. For example, sometimes people new to clinical supervision are disturbed and even angry that complete confidentiality cannot be promised, and careful reference to the codes which people profess will help in showing that this is not possible. You will be able to think of other examples.

✐ Your thoughts

What other areas of conflict may arise from differences in codes of practice?

Other issues

The giving and receiving of **feedback** is an essential part of clinical supervision. After all, there is little point in the activity if there is no exchange of ideas or opinions! Clinical supervision's formative function is educative and developmental, and feedback plays an important role in this. The contract should make clear that feedback is (like confidentiality) a mutual activity. The supervisor is not a teacher giving instruction – the 'mug and jug' model, where the 'mug' (the supervisee) is receiving information from the 'jug' (the supervisor), is not appropriate in this context. The supervisor should be as open to receiving feedback as to giving it. As well as being part of every session in the normal 'give and take' of the process, feedback is also part of the reviewing process: from time to time (possibly at agreed intervals) it is very helpful to step back and consider how the work is going and where it might go in the future.

Reviewing helps to keep the aims of the clinical supervision work in focus, perhaps by using the formative, normative, restorative, and perspective categories as points of reference. Referring to the four functions can also serve as a reminder, indicating whether there has been appropriate balance in the sessions. This is what one supervisor said about her first experience:

👁 **Witness statement**

Reviewing was a good lesson for me. I realised that we had spent far too long working on his dissatisfactions, which I suppose was restorative in a way, but it also meant that we didn't do enough about how he could set about putting things right, although I knew that what he and probably his whole team really needed was some training. Once I woke up to that through the review, I was able to give him some feedback and he went off to look for suitable courses and to find out how to access funding.

Take each of the four functions and suggest some disadvantages that may arise if there is too much emphasis on one single area. For example, too much time spent on the restorative element could mean that the relationship is slipping into personal (or peer) counselling.

✍ **Your thoughts**

What problems could arise if there is over-emphasis in a particular function?

- Formative
- Normative
- Restorative
- Perspective

Establishing a contract which covers all these issues, yet does not threaten the supervisee, is a very skilful task. It can require communication skills of a high order.

Once the contract has been agreed, the supervisor will work to build and maintain the supervisory relationship. Try to answer the following questions:

✍ **Your thoughts**

1. Why do you want to be a clinical supervisor?
2. Do you think you will be a good clinical supervisor? Why?

cont../.

> 3. What relevant skills do you already have?
> 4. What skills do you need to develop?

Let's consider each of these in turn.

1. One very good reason for wanting to be a clinical supervisor is because you believe that supervision can make a difference to the supervisee by encouraging reflective practice, which should in turn facilitate his or her professional growth and development (and often personal development too). Another good reason is that the patient receiving palliative care and the organisation providing it will receive discernible benefits.

2. The second question is not so easy to answer. Carers, by their nature, seem to be reluctant to praise themselves! But you yourself may have felt that your own practice would benefit if there were a safe forum for discussion. Perhaps you have realised that your colleagues would benefit from the sort of clinical supervision you have been fortunate enough to receive and would like to replicate it for them. Perhaps you think (and it is not immodest to do so!) That you possess the qualities that we explored in *Chapter Two*.

3. Many of the interpersonal or basic counselling skills are used by palliative care practitioners in their day-to-day communication with patients and colleagues. Ways of giving help can be represented as a continuum – at one end of the spectrum the helper is pro-active, doing things for or on behalf of another; and moving along the spectrum increasingly more responsibility is given to the person being helped.

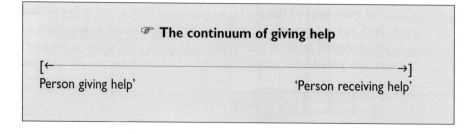

☞ **The continuum of giving help**

[← ————————————————————————— →]
Person giving help'   'Person receiving help'

Every task on the continuum of giving help is enhanced by the use of good communication skills (see *Figure 4.1.*)

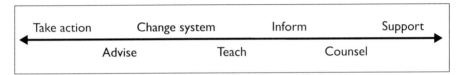

Figure 4.1: The helping continuum

In the early stages of being a clinical supervisor, many practitioners find it difficult to use appropriate challenge. They need to develop this skill, because challenge is an essential part of the analysis and feedback of which the process is composed. Often there are concerns that challenge will somehow damage the working alliance, but without challenge (given responsibly) there is a danger of collusion.

Communicating in clinical supervision

One of the qualities you may have identified about yourself in response to the second and third questions is being a good listener. There is no doubt that being listened to is something that supervisees truly value. It is consistently rated very highly in surveys of what supervisees find most helpful in their supervisor. This knowledge may, sadly, reflect the fact that too often in our work *we* do not feel really listened to, despite the fact that we spend a great deal of time spent listening to patients or bereaved people as part of our palliative care commitment. Not being heard is not good for morale, and it will affect job satisfaction at some point. (It is interesting to note that not being listened to is frequently a complaint made by patients too – perhaps you can provide some examples).

✎ **Your thoughts**

What situations can you think of in which we do not listen to patients enough?

Listening is a complex activity, which can be very tiring. Its complexity means that if we are listening fully we need to:

- focus solely on the speaker
- take in the whole message
- sustain the focus
- hear feelings as well as content
- listen to the person as well as to the 'problem'.

In addition we need to 'listen' with our eyes, so to speak, as well as with our ears – how does the person look? Are there any changes? What's happening with their body language? This special form of listening which supervisors need to develop is usually termed **active listening** and has been called 'the most effective form of communication' (Hough, 1998). The skill of active listening is often underestimated and the degree of effort it involves is not always appreciated.

Read the following scenario which has been adapted from a group clinical supervision session in a hospice. The work being discussed concerns a relative of a palliative care patient, who was very distressed at what she saw as her mother's (the patient's) rejection.

◉ Witness statement

Hospice social worker She apologises time and time again for going over and over the same ground, but she clearly finds it very distressing that her mother turns her head away every time she tries to kiss her goodbye.

Clinical supervisor Could you tell us what you said to her.

Social worker We-ell... I tried to help her get some sort of balance and pointed out that she had often told me that her mother never was one for showing her affection physically. I'd noticed myself that she isn't very tactile – never returns a squeeze of the hand – and I mentioned this.

Clinical supervisor Could I throw that open. Is that OK? [social worker nods] Would anyone else have handled her distress in a different way?

Hospice nurse [tentatively] I'm not really sure, but I might have tried to empathise with her distress. When you told us that she said, 'It's so hurtful that she turns away my affection', what came into my mind was 'That sounds like real grief for you'. So I might have said something like that. I don't know if it would have helped her any better.

✐ **Your thoughts**

Which of the two responses do you think showed *active* listening, and why?

I would say that although the social worker had heard the *factual* content of the daughter's concern she had missed the *emotional* content, and by assuming that what was needed was reassurance she had given her own interpretation of the mother's behaviour rather than hearing the daughter's distress. (The supervisor went on to open up the discussion with other members of the team, very carefully ensuring that there was no criticism and that the social worker was able to reflect on whether the feedback had been useful.)

So, in addition to the aspects of listening already mentioned, we have to be aware of our own feelings as well as those of the other person. A palliative care patient once described to me how awkward he had felt when he came round from an anaesthetic after an amputation to find care staff holding his hands, and expecting him to be very emotional.

👁 **Witness statement**

In fact, all I felt was relief, and I didn't know what to do since they were obviously geared up to cope with tears or rage, or something. I think I was more responsible for their distress than they were for me!

Keeping our own feelings in check and not assuming that others will feel as we do is also part of active listening.

I wonder who it was who suggested that listening is a simple activity?! Its complexity is awe inspiring. Complex or not, many palliative care practitioners possess the skill at a high level and use it more or less unconsciously with their patients. The skill is equally valuable in a supervisor, despite the different nature of the relationship. The supervisory relationship may be quite therapeutic for both parties, but it is not therapy, and so the use of active listening is for a rather different purpose.

Compare these two scenarios. In both situations a hospice nurse is the listener. In the first she is talking with a patient in palliative care. In the second she is the clinical supervisor of a hospice volunteer home visitor.

◉ **Witness statements**

Scenario 1

Patient I'm so tired. I just don't feel I can fight any more. I know it distresses him if I say I've had enough, but it's the truth.

Nurse You sound exhausted and it's almost as if you wish your husband would somehow give you permission to end the struggle?

Patient Yes. It's not that I want euthanasia or whatever you call it, just that he'd let me go. When I try to say goodbye and thank you he seems so scared. So I never get to say what I need to.

Nurse You seem very sad. You don't want to hurry the end, but at the same time your compassion for — makes the final break hard for you, which isn't how you want it to be.

Scenario 2

Volunteer I'm at a bit of a loss really. I go in there to sit, you know, and give the wife a bit of respite, but it doesn't seem to work.

Nurse Can you explain that a bit? What exactly doesn't work? You seem a bit fed up about it.

Volunteer Well, to start with, she won't leave us when the whole point is to give her a little break, but she's in and out with cups of tea and chat about this and that. It's a waste of time.

Nurse We may need to come back to that comment about waste of time, but tell me first what else doesn't seem to work.

Volunteer Hmmm... When she's out of the room, he either doesn't seem to want me there, turns the TV on or something, or starts to whisper and then stops the minute she returns with cake and stuff – and it's very embarrassing. She must wonder about secrets or if I'm colluding with him in some way.

Nurse Can I sum up what you've said so far. You're feeling frustrated because the work you thought you were there to do doesn't seem to be wanted and at the same time maybe worried that there's some kind of agenda with the patient that you just don't 'get'.

Volunteer Yes, that's about it. Do you think I should stop going?

Nurse Let's have a look at what you've achieved so far and then have a think about what you might do to confront the situation. Then maybe you'll be able to make a decision about the best way forward for all of you.

In both her roles the nurse is certainly being empathic and in neither case does she shirk her responsibility – she does not ignore the patient's wish to die nor try to distract her onto a different line of thought; she does not tell the volunteer what to do, but offers to work *with* him to come to some sort of resolution. It is especially interesting that with the volunteer she does not get diverted into talking about the patient and the patient's wife, but stays firmly focused on his work *with* the couple. This is a critical skill for supervisors. Here, it would be very easy (and interesting) to ask for details about the couple and about their relationship (and a few details may become necessary for the sake of clarity) but the focus of clinical supervision is on the practitioner's work with patients or clients – not the patients or clients themselves (important though they are). Both scenarios are good examples of active listening, and both demonstrate that vital quality of empathy (Carl Rogers, 1975).

> *Empathy is the ability to experience another person's world as if it were one's own without losing the 'as if'.*

In a sense, however, the listening and the empathy are used to achieve both similar and different aims. The interaction with the patient aims to deepen rapport and to facilitate, perhaps clarify, the patient's emotions and concerns; similarly, the nurse supervisor is sensitive to the volunteer's emotions (noting that he is 'a bit fed up' and 'frustrated' and 'worried') and she is working towards gaining clarification. The difference is that she has no intention to 'solve' any of the patient's problems (that is, her approach is not solution-focused) whereas in the volunteer interaction she is solution focused. Here we can clearly see the difference between counselling and supervision. The process of clinical supervision should provide a sort of containment or 'holding' environment so that supervisees are encouraged to express their feelings about their work. But that is not its chief function. The supervision work may well help the volunteer's feelings as part of its restorative function (and it's interesting that the nurse mentions achievements as the basis for the next step in their discussion) but its main focus is on the volunteer's *work*, not on him himself. It is also worth noting the skills that the nurse uses:

- With the patient she uses reflection, advanced empathy and summary.
- With the volunteer she uses open questions and focusing ('concreteness').
- In both roles the nurse needed to develop trust. Once again this is a two-way process. That the supervisee needs to trust the supervisor almost goes without saying, but it would be helpful in terms of self-awareness to list the ways in which your supervisee (or a potential supervisee) could trust you.

Trust and challenge

You have now considered the issues of confidentiality, of being non-judgemental, and many of the other qualities we explored in *Chapter Two*. Of course being trustworthy and confident in your own trustworthiness is one thing – ensuring that a supervisee knows and believes that you are may be another thing altogether! Try to keep a diary of ways in which you can demonstrate your trustworthiness so that you develop your supervisees' trust in you as a clinical supervisor. One way of doing this is to maximise opportunities for working in a non-hierarchical way. Another is to model how the supervisee will take responsibility for using clinical supervision to the best advantage.

Consider the following statement by Proctor (1991):

It is a fantasy that I as a supervisor can gain access by demand to what is essentially a private relationship. In reality the work people do with other people is predominantly 'unsupervised'. What someone brings to supervision is selective and subject to 'presentation'. What is watched or heard direct (or on video or audiotape) is always partial and influenced by the watching or hearing. I can encourage my supervisee to give me more appropriate access to her practice. I cannot control the courage, honesty, good will or perception which determine the presentation (or performance) she chooses to give me.

Realistically, even the supervisee's choice of what to bring to clinical supervision to work on will depend on the degree of trust in the relationship.

Offering someone the opportunity to analyse and comment on one's work takes courage, and supervisees will not disclose in any depth unless there is trust. Part of building the supervisory relationship and developing the working alliance involves nurturing trust. The supervisor therefore needs to look for opportunities to demonstrate trustworthiness.

When trust is established (not that it is a fixed, unchanging quality) the supervisor may find opportunities for challenge. Many supervisors, especially those new to the task are wary of challenging their supervisees. Having worked hard to build a trusting and mutual alliance, they are concerned that challenge may destroy it. The term 'challenge' is often interpreted as 'confrontation' and it presents the same sort of difficulties as the word 'supervision.' The problem is that all too often confrontation is used as accusation, and as a way of off-loading irritations or other negative emotions ('just look what you've done!' Or 'oh no – you didn't do that!') – But responsible challenge is an important component of feedback and when used well it can really help to enhance practice.

Work through the following questions as honestly as you can and reflect on whether you need to think about how to use appropriate challenge as a supervisor.

✐ Your thoughts

When were you challenged and able to use that challenge to improve yourself (perhaps to improve your practice)?
When have you received challenge and found it too hurtful to be of use? Was it hurtful at the time? Since? What was the difference?
Do you ever enjoy challenging someone?
Do you think that you challenge in such a way that others accept it?
Do you avoid challenging or put it off for as long as possible? If so, what is your concern?

Loyalty to patients should mean that any malpractice is challenged, and some kind of action or way forward is agreed. Thankfully, the need to challenge malpractice or bad practice is very rare in the palliative care field (and a practitioner capable of it is unlikely to be using clinical supervision appropriately anyway), but there are issues and interventions that a supervisor could challenge which would encourage reflective practice. Enquiring why a specific intervention was made is not accusation or criticism, but an invitation to consider the rationale and perhaps to explore alternatives.

Gerard Egan, who has written extensively on 'helping', and whose phase model of helping could be as useful for supervisors as it is for counsellors or others using counselling skills to enhance their work has offered some helpful comments about challenge (Egan, 1999).

Support without challenge is hollow; challenge without support can be abrasive.

Take a moment to write down what you think Egan meant.

✏ **Your thoughts**

What did Egan mean by his comments on support and challenge?

If we apply that statement to clinical supervision we will need first of all to agree that the supervision process is supportive. It's unfortunate that the word 'supportive' has been so over-used that it has lost the full force of its meaning. Remind yourself (again!) Of the formative, normative, restorative, and perspective functions of clinical supervision. Would you see each function as 'supportive'? In what way or ways?

✏ **Your thoughts**

How is each of these functions 'supportive'?

- Formative
- Normative
- Restorative
- Perspective

Egan seems to be saying that if there is no challenge in the support it can be rather bland or empty. Sometimes the supervisory relationship can become too 'cosy'. There is particular risk of this happening in peer supervision, where the participants know each other and have their work and their patients and clients in common. There is a tendency for discussion of cases and caseloads and commiseration with each other's difficulties to take the place of supervision. On the other hand, Egan points out that challenge without support is likely to result in conflict, and sometimes hurt feelings.

Here is what a member of a palliative care team in a children's hospice said.

◉ Witness statement

Eventually I had to ask for a different clinical supervisor, even though I liked her enormously. The trouble was that I never felt that I was going anywhere. She praised everything that I did, which of course was nice (and I needed it because my line manager was a bit mean with praise!) but it was always the same. Sort of 'Tell me what you did' followed by blanket approval. I remember I was really stuck about one family and she empathised with my 'stuck-ness' but that's as far as it went... when what I needed was some suggestions for looking at things differently. The person I'm with now pushes me to look at how I'm working and whether I could do anything differently. It's pretty tiring sometimes, but I do think I'm *moving* even if I don't always know where!

Egan also says that we have to 'earn the right' to challenge. He suggests that we earn that right by being prepared to be challenged ourselves. This is very pertinent for clinical supervision because if there is genuine mutuality in the relationship and it is a true working alliance then the supervisee should be able to use challenge reciprocally.

It may be easier to appreciate the concept of the skill of challenge as appropriate and reciprocal if we see the participants as challenging *issues* rather than *persons* and as a way of facilitating development.

What follows are the words of a new clinical supervisor.

◉ Witness statement

Even after training, I still somehow thought that *I* had to be the fount of all knowledge (as if!). And I was worried about what would happen if my supervisee challenged me about anything. I didn't want to be defensive, but I was nervous. Actually, it worked out well, because after we'd analysed some of the interventions she's made, she asked me 'What would you have done?' and I was able to reflect and share with her my likely actions *and* to say that I

cont../.

---

thought hers were probably more effective in that situation. Then we went on to look at whether there were any other possibilities. I have to say, though, that I don't think I could have achieved that if we hadn't had a contract, which made me confident that she wouldn't use challenge to undermine me in any way.

That witness statement partially illustrates another point that Egan makes about earning the right to challenge. He thinks that we should be constantly challenging ourselves. Using the four functions as a basis, check whether you could challenge yourself.

✐ Your thoughts

Formative
Do your skills need developing in any way?
How often do you take time to reflect on your practice?
Have you broadened your understanding of palliative care?
What new knowledge are you acquiring about palliative care?
How do you respond to issues raised by your patients/clients/colleagues/supervisees?
Normative
If asked, could you explain the ethics of your profession as they relate to palliative care?
What do you know about the standards and ethics of the agency you're involved with (eg. hospice, NHS, Macmillan, Marie Curie, other)?
How is your own practice monitored?
Is there any system for receiving feedback on your practice? Do you or could you act on it?
Restorative
Do you have a safe forum where you can deal with personal issues and stresses arising from your palliative care work?
Do you ever give yourself a pat on the back?
Perspective
How good an overview do you have of your total caseload/work?
Are you able to articulate the relationship between your own practice and other ways in which patients and clients could receive help?
What is your relationship with co-practitioners? Could you improve it?
What is your relationship with members of other relevant professions? Should you extend it?

Since helping with these issues (and many others) comprise the service that supervisors hope to offer supervisees, it reinforces a recommendation that:

Supervisors require opportunity for supervision themselves to sustain them in their role.

The importance of balancing support and challenge cannot be overstated. Indeed getting the balance right is one of the most critical supervisor skills. It involves, of course, giving feedback. The basic skills 'tool kit' for conducting a supervision session consists of:

- paraphrasing
- reflecting
- appropriate questioning
- summarising
- 'teaching' (in the sense of sharing knowledge).

All these could come under the heading of 'feedback'.

Feedback

Here are some guidelines for giving feedback, adapted from a book by the British Association for Counselling and Psychotherapy *Counselling Skills in Context* (BACP, 2001).

☞ **A guide to giving feedback**

Give specific and accurate feedback. Where feedback is negative, suggest alternatives and remember feedback says at least as much about the giver as the receiver.

1. Offer feedback on observed behaviour, not on perceived attitudes.
2. Offer a description of what you heard and how you felt, rather than a judgement.
3. Focus on anything which might be changed.
4, Choose which aspects are most important and limit yourself to those.
5. Ask genuine questions. (This is a good way to practise how to use questions without manipulation.)

cont../.

---

6. Make statements which involve owning your responsibility, such as 'I'd experienced you as —'
7. Set the ground rules in advance.
8. Comment on the things that an individual did well, as well as areas for improvement.
9. Relate all your feedback to specific items of behaviour rather than general failings or impressions ('When you said — the client seems to have —').
10. Observe everyone's personal limits – not too much feedback at once.
11. Before offering any feedback, consider its value for the receiver.

Adapted from BACP (2001).

Try to get some feedback on the way you give feedback (the triad model is useful for this).

Structuring the clinical supervision session is also a good skill to acquire and practise. Here is a list of suggestions of how a session might be structured.

1. The agenda for the supervision session is agreed at the beginning of each session. Timing is negotiated.
2. Supervisees are facilitated in identifying their developmental needs and opportunities through regularly reviewing the process and use made of supervision.
3. Opportunities are provided for the exploration, accommodation and use of the supervisee's responses and reactions to clients and patients.
4. Supervisees are encouraged to identify their practice issues and areas for improvement.
5. Supervisees are facilitated in exploring ways in which theories of palliative care inform practice.
6. Relationship issues and processes are used as material for the exploration of the supervisee's work.
7. Supervisees are encouraged to examine the relevance and relationship between the supervisory process and their own work with patients and clients.
8. The process of supervision is regularly evaluated and appropriate adjustments made.

✐ **Your thoughts**

Try to make an evaluative comment for each item on the preceding list.

Additionally, it may be good to ensure that:

- The way in which supervisees operate their agreed ethical code is clearly identified, evidenced and monitored.
- Management of caseload is regularly reviewed and monitored to ensure effectiveness and competence.
- Good practice and new learning is recognised, acknowledged and validated.
- Evidence of 'not good enough' practice (if identified) is constructively challenged and ways of remedying it are explored and monitored.
- Information and help is offered if supervisees appear to be reaching burn out.
- Consultation is sought if obstacles, difficulties arise in the working alliance.

There is evidence that 'structure' is in itself helpful, so it is worthwhile for the supervisor to look at these points and to work out the order for covering them that would best suit the supervisor and the supervisee. Making sure that there is an identifiable 'shape' to the sessions will enhance their effectiveness.

From time to time, the clinical supervision needs an overall review, so time should be set aside to consider and evaluate:

- How clinical supervision is affecting the supervisee's practice.
- Whether the supervisee's goals and expectations of clinical supervision are being met.
- How much learning for both parties has been achieved.
- The nature of the caseload.
- Any adjustments that may be needed (to the contract or to the relationship, for example)

This chapter has concentrated on the role and skills of the supervisor, but of course the success or otherwise of clinical supervision depends equally upon the supervisee and this role is what we look at in *Chapter Five* – remembering that supervisors also need supervision, and so are themselves potential supervisees.

References

BACP (2001) *Counselling Skills in Context* British Association for Counselling and Psychotherapy, Rugby

BACP (1996) *Code of Ethics and Practice for Supervisors of Counsellors*. British Association for Counselling and Psychotherapy, Rugby.

BACP (2001) *Ethical Framework for Good Practice in Counselling and Psychotherapy*. BACP, Rugby

Butterworth T, Carson J, White E, Jeacock J, Clements A, Bishop V (1997) *It Is Good To Talk: An Evaluation Study of Clinical Supervision in England and Scotland*. University of Manchester, Manchester

Cook DA, Helms JE (1988) Visible racial/ethnic group supervisees' satisfaction with cross-cultural supervision as predicted by relationship characteristics. *J Counseling Psychol* **35**(3): 268–274

Egan G (1999) *The Skilled Helper*. Brookes Cole, California

Hough M (1998) *Counselling Skills and Theory*. Hodder and Stoughton, London

Proctor B (1991) Supervision: a co-operative exercise in accountability. In: Marken M, Payne M (eds) *Enabling and Ensuring Supervision in Practice*. National Youth Bureau, Leicester

Rogers CR (1975) Empathic: an unappreciated way of being. *The Councelling Psychologist* **2**: 2–10

CHAPTER 5

Being a supervisee

Clinical supervision involves at least two people, face to face, with the 'shadowy' presence of a third person – the patient, client or colleague around whom the supervisee's concerns revolve. In the previous chapter we stressed that clinical supervision is not a one-way relationship, but a working alliance in which there are equal (albeit different) contributions from each party. This is partly exemplified by the non-managerial, non-hierarchical nature of the relationship. The supervisee is an equal and active partner in the process, so being clear, as supervisees, about what we want from our own clinical supervision and how our contribution can help to achieve our goals is vital for success.

Here is a list (in no particular order) of what practitioners in palliative care have said that they want from clinical supervision. Check whether the list resonates with your own wants or needs, and add any points you might see as necessary.

☞ **What practitioners want from clinical supervision**

Practitioners want:
- Periodic review of personal and professional progress
- Alternative things to say or do
- Encouragement and support
- Guidance about style
- Safety (emotional and physical) of clients, patients and self
- A watch on the overall caseload and working conditions
- Teaching/guidance about new thinking in palliative care
- To know how to link up with other providers or alternative help
- Help with personal issues (eg if they really can't get on with someone)
- Contact in an emergency
- Ethical guidance
- To know what to do about spiritual issues
- Insight into palliative care with patients and clients from other ethnic or cultural backgrounds

cont../.

- Monitoring of personal and professional development (which is different from 'progress')
- Guidance about books or relevant articles
- Understanding of their nervousness about clinical supervision
- Confidentiality
- Challenge
- A widening of their range of skills and techniques
- Advice
- Help with identifying dynamics (between self and patients, colleagues, and supervisor)

You might find it helpful to go through the list again and write F, N, R, or P against each item, to show whether it seems to be a request for help on Formative, Normative, Restorative or Perspective functions.

Identifying the nature of the clinical supervision you require will help you to seek out the most appropriate supervision and supervisor for you. Of course, this may not always be possible; some organisations allocate supervisors to supervisees and vice versa, perhaps because they are thought to be 'good' for each other, or because of availability. Time constraints and timetabling may make this sort of allocation inevitable. Even so, identifying needs, wants, and expectations will make the task of contracting much more focused. To identify the type of clinical supervision you hope for, it's useful to take into account the range or variety of your current patients or clients and the range of therapeutic activity you are engaged in with them. You might also like to reflect on what stage you think you are at with regard to your personal competence and your professional development.

The box below shows what a hospice education officer said on the matter.

◉ Witness statement

Since I had come into the job from being a Macmillan nurse, I thought that my practical skills were pretty up to date, and that as I was teaching courses on them I had to keep them that way! On the other hand, I was at zero level with my teaching and management skills. In a way, my 'clients' were the students, but I am also a member of the palliative care team. So I thought it would be difficult to find a clinical supervisor, but my manager suggested the hospice counsellor and that worked well, because he could question me because *he* needed clarification about some aspects of my work and that helped me to clarify.

This person had anticipated difficulty in finding suitable clinical supervision. If you are fortunate enough to have a choice, you will evaluate the available options, taking account of:

- clinical focus (where you hope for support and challenge)
- the professional monitoring of your practice
- your professional development
- your learning needs
- the repertoire of skills you have and those you need to develop
- choices that are open to you for development (personal and professional).

Using these points, try to identify where you might find clinical supervision that meets the criteria, or other criteria which you might have for yourself. Does it exist within your organisation or might you have to seek it from an outside source?

✐ Your thoughts

Where might you find clinical supervision that meets the criteria above (or any criteria of your own)?

The contract

If you are then fortunate enough to be able to choose a supervisor, you would probably need to consider how congruent she or he is with your own ethical stance and approach to palliative care. You might ask yourself whether he or she (however much you respect them) is appropriate for your current work and for the level of expertise that you have. Respecting your clinical supervisor will perhaps also involve consideration of their experience and expertise as a supervisor (not necessarily as a palliative care practitioner). It is, however, worth noting that where clinical supervision is new to an organisation both parties may, so to speak, be learning on the job. This is especially likely if peer supervision is the preferred model.

Go through that list again and reflect on whether you now feel ready to make a clinical supervision contract.

As we indicated in *Chapter Four* many people who are new to clinical supervision are very nervous of the term 'contract'. Just as 'supervision' may have unfortunate undertones, so 'contract' may sound too formal or legalistic. I was once asked: 'If I agree to this contract is it legally binding?'.

The object of the contract is not to tie people down – especially not to tie down supervisees – but to ensure that both parties have agreed some ground rules. This facilitates the process of clinical supervision and ensures the mutuality that is so vital for the working alliance. It goes without saying that the supervisor should not impose the 'conditions' of the contract, and there will be no danger of this if supervisees take the responsibility for being clear about what they want and need and expect.

Here is what two very well-known writers (Hawkins and Shohet, 1989) said about supervision:

> *To ensure nurses get the supervision they want, they must take full responsibility; contracting and negotiating how this supervision will operate and how it will be monitored and reviewed.*

Do you agree? Why? Why not? As a potential supervisee, you will want to clarify the practical details of your clinical supervision. Such details would include:

- The time, place, and arrangements for contact (should appointments have to be missed, or in case of a crisis, for example).
- Arrangements for record taking and record keeping.
- The possibility of payment (your supervisor may be paid by your organisation and have obligations because of this, which you might want to clarify; any third party involvement could affect the supervisory relationship in a number of ways).
- What might happen if your practice is seen as not 'good enough'.
- Confidentiality and other boundaries.
- What you hope to gain from clinical supervision.

You may also want your contract to be explicit about each of your roles, your joint responsibilities, your obligations and commitments. Accountability may mean different things to different people or different organisations: your supervisor may be accountable both to you and to your organisation. You yourself are likely to be responsible to your supervisor, your organisation, your line manager, or your professional body if you have one. Ultimately all parties in clinical supervision are accountable to patients and clients. If these issues are clarified in the contract, it will help to set the relationship off on an open footing and will engender trust.

Write down your personal aims and objectives for clinical supervision.

✎ **Your thoughts**

What are your personal aims and objectives for clinical supervision?

Your list might have included these points:

- self-monitoring
- monitoring of your work to ensure that it is benefiting your patients and clients
- your personal and professional development
- your on-going education
- extension of your knowledge and skills.

Sometimes a clinical supervision contract sets out an agreement about ways of working. Some of the issues that are considered if this is part of the agreement are listed below.

- Whether there is congruence between the supervisor's ethical code and your own.
- How to monitor the boundary between 'training' and 'development' (clinical supervision is educational, but it is not a training course).
- How to maintain the non-managerial, non-hierarchical nature of the relationship.
- The nature of what issues will be brought for supervision work.
- The balance of challenge and support.

Now try now to write a contract that you think you could agree with a supervisor, and which you would see as a sound basis for a working alliance.

✎ **Your thoughts**

What should the supervisor–supervisee contract contain?

The working alliance

In the working alliance, one of the supervisee's responsibilities is to select appropriate material for supervision work.

A supervisee who was undertaking post-qualifying training for palliative care wrote: 'I took — to supervision.' Her supervisor wrote in the margin 'I don't think we take our patients to supervision – we take ourselves.' What is your view about this?

✐ **Your thoughts**

Exactly who takes whom to supervision?

I think perhaps the supervisor was trying to convey two things:

Firstly, (as the book has stressed throughout), that clinical supervision is not about patients or clients but about the supervisee's work with them. As Supervisees we should be constantly asking ourselves:

- What am I doing with this patient/client now? This minute?
- Why am I doing it?

Secondly, that to reflect on our work we need to reflect on ourselves and ask:

- How well do I think I'm doing?
- What am I finding good/bad about my work?
- What skills do I need to develop?
  (These are just a few of the possibilities!)

Here is an exercise that has been found helpful in preparation for supervision and for deciding what material you wish to focus on. You need to set aside about ten minutes when you can be quiet and free from interruptions. It is useful to have a note pad to hand.

✐ Your thoughts

Part One

Let your mind drift back over your palliative care work of the past week (or few weeks).

■ What stood out? Remember it.
■ What are you pleased with?

Remember interventions, actions, exchanges that went well. Recall what was difficult. Some decisions may have been hard to make; some patients or their relatives may have presented you with difficult choices; there may have been issues or conflict with colleagues.

■ Are you unsure about any decisions you made (even though they were made in good faith)?
■ What anxieties (if any) do you have about your work with particular patients/clients?
■ Are there any tensions with colleagues?
■ Is there something you'd prefer not to disclose to your supervisor? Try to identify why.
■ What are you looking forward to in your next week's/month's work?

Part Two

Now make a brief list of what cropped up as you were reflecting. On your list, highlight the items that seem worth discussing in clinical supervision (if you leave out any items, check with yourself why you have omitted them).

■ Prioritise the items on the list.
■ Decide what you want to learn in supervision from discussing those priorities.
■ Decide how you will present your material.

In *Chapter Four* you read about how reliant a supervisor can be on what a supervisee chooses to offer, and on how the material is presented. The supervisor thus must *trust* the supervisee, and we need to bear this in mind when we are preparing for sessions. The degree of trust will of course depend, to some extent, on the supervisor and nature of the working alliance, but once again the mutuality (in this case a mutuality of trust) is paramount.

The success of the actual clinical supervision session will be enhanced by sound preparation. The way in which the session is structured is also crucial to its success and does not depend solely on the supervisor – if it does there is probably something amiss, as both parties should be taking responsibility for the process as well as the content of the session. Here are some suggestions as guidelines for a successful clinical supervision session:

- It is helpful to start by negotiating the content and agenda with the supervisor. Just as with any meeting, having a list of items you want to explore will help the focus.
- As supervisee, you will have prepared the material beforehand (although your supervisor may also wish to bring forward items), and it is the supervisee's responsibility to organise, manage and present the material clearly.
- Bearing in mind the four elements of supervision, a supervisee should be able to recognise which aspects of the material require supervisory attention. These might include: therapeutic relationships; processes; activities; ethical issues; theoretical issues; issues evoked in you by patients/clients and the nature of the work; casework management; technical competence; your own physical, mental or emotional state; mistakes or difficult moments; blocks to progress; successes.
- Be open about any anxieties about clinical supervision in order to engage in non-defensive reflection as a result of feedback. Some of these anxieties may centre around the power issues we discussed earlier or about fears of not being in control; some supervisees are over-anxious to impress or to please the supervisor.
- Question and challenge the supervisor in order to gain from his or her expertise.
- Relate feedback to practical management of the case work and to further one's own progress and development.

Working through a structure of this kind will help a supervisee to the gain most from the session.

In terms of **self-awareness** it is important to recognise and acknowledge feelings about clinical supervision and about one's supervisor, and might include the following:

- Your professional competence and its limitations.
- Your responses to difficulties and your feelings about disclosing these in clinical supervision.
- Your personal feelings about your supervisor and the help he or she is offering.
- Any potential blocks you may be experiencing about making the best use of supervision.
- Your personal needs and whether you think they are being met.

Being aware of these feelings will help to ensure that they do not become a barrier to either the working alliance or to personal and professional progress and development. An awareness of feelings will also encourage a supervisee's ability to question and challenge appropriately as a tool for his or her own development, and to really use feedback to enhance reflective practice.

Supervisee competence

In *Chapter Five* we mentioned levels of supervisee competence. There has been great use of the **four levels of supervisee competence** originally proposed by Francesca Inskipp (1998) and now seemingly in general use. These are used as the basis of the discussion that follows. The level the practitioner is at will affect how the supervisor works and at what depth. It will also affect the process of their relationship.

Here is what two palliative care practitioners said when clinical supervision was first introduced into their unit (attached to a small community hospital).

◉ Witness statements

First practitioner Although I had been nursing for quite some time I was new to palliative care, and even though I'd achieved the qualification I knew that I still had a great deal to learn. There was great morale in the team, but I still felt anxious... always nervous in case I didn't get things right. I really needed help, but I didn't want to lose face!

Second practitioner I had a lot of palliative care experience. I'd worked on an oncology ward and then in two hospices, one a hospice-at-home and one with a bedded unit for inpatient provision. BUT I had never had the type of clinical supervision they introduced. I expected it to be either case discussion, or a sort of managerial overseeing, only not with my line manager. As you can hear, I may have known a lot about palliative care, but I was a novice about non-managerial supervision (just as well they didn't ask me to be a supervisor then – I'd have been useless!).

As you read now about the four suggested levels (which have been adapted considerably from the original) try to gauge your own level of competence.

First level of practice

This level is supervisee centred. Practitioners tend to be very dependent on the supervisor, and to seek mainly advice and guidance. They tend to be anxious about ability and suitability for the work. This may be very prevalent in palliative care because the change from cure goals to care goals can be very profound for those new to the profession. The nature of the work – collaborative, following the patient, focusing on quality of life for the patient through to death, and often care of the bereaved relatives – presents a huge challenge for all of us and those new to it may feel very insecure. The first-level supervisee may also be concerned (sometimes over-concerned) about what other team members and line managers may be expecting.

An experienced practitioner new to clinical supervision may share some of these tendencies, and this is why getting a really sound contract in place is crucial.

✎ Your thoughts

How does your own level of competence compare with the first level of practice?

Second level of practice

At this level the supervisee is more patient- or client-focused. As they progresses in palliative care and become increasingly involved with the work, the supervisee will tend to seek ideas and information of a practical nature in relation to patients. In palliative care this may be about drugs, diet, or symptoms. You can see how this could make the peer or same-discipline models useful. On the other hand, this kind of advice may be better sought from a line manager. It is at this level, too, that the supervisee may oscillate between over-involvement with a patient/client and distance from a patient/client, and this would be a very appropriate area for supervision. As clinical supervision progresses there should be a growth in the ability to analyse interactions and processes and to see how the dynamic of these affects the work. It may be very helpful to discuss the effect that working with the dynamic has on the supervisee's confidence about the more practical areas of work.

✐ Your thoughts

How does your own level of competence compare with the second level of practice?

Third level of practice

As the supervisee's professional competence increases, self-confidence grows. The supervisee is much more able to analyse and make sense of palliative care in terms of interactions with patients, clients and relatives, rather than by focusing on the practical helping skills, essential though these are. There is less preoccupation with what to *do* for people and more interest in how to *be* with them. Supervisees begin to be able to think about the people they work to help and about themselves in terms of systems – cultural, family, and organisational. In palliative care this has a special resonance, as the network of family and others (which may not always impact on the work in the way one might hope) is a crucial factor. Similarly, palliative care is a multi-professional approach to people at an exceptionally vulnerable time and supervisees at this level begin to see themselves and their work in terms of the system they are in, rather than seeing things as solely to do with themselves and their patients. In other words, they grow more aware of the process of their work rather than of the content.

A sense of greater colleagueship with the supervisor is likely to develop as their working relationship deepens and this may lead to helpful ways of challenging the supervisor and to the use of challenge as a tool for challenging his or her own practice. This growing confidence is often signalled by the supervisee's ability to discriminate about appropriate aspects of work for supervision focus.

📎 **Your thoughts**

How does your own level of competence compare with the third level of practice?

Fourth level of practice

By now, the mutuality of the working alliance should be firmly established. The supervisee may well be supervising others, and learning from this is an additional way for supervisees to develop their own education (in the broadest sense of the word) and practice. Supervisees at this level are very clear are about their own wants and needs in relation to clinical supervision. The non-hierarchical nature of the supervisory relationship should be very clear. Each session should show that both the content and process of clinical supervision has been reflected on and used to inform aspects of patient or client work – and this should be true for both parties. There may well be signs that the supervisee is seeking further training – a thirst for greater knowledge and understanding is the bonus of good clinical supervision.

📎 **Your thoughts**

How does your own level of competence compare with the fourth level of practice?

Although this chapter focuses on the supervisee there are clearly implications for how a supervisor will work at each level and what skills he or she will need to further the working alliance. In the box below, try to list what skills a supervisor would need at each level to ensure that clinical supervision (not for instance case discussion or counselling) is taking place.

✎ **Your thoughts**

What skills are needed by a supervisor to ensure that clinical supervision is taking place?

- At level one?
- At level two?
- At level three?
- At level four?

Your suggestions may have included:

Level one
- Basic active listening to explore the supervisee's issues.
- Use of empathy to lay the foundation for the working relationship.
- Frequent referral to the boundary issues agreed in the contract.

Level two
- Choosing between being an 'educator' and on concentrating on emotional issues.
- Developing the practitioner's ability to learn and understand for themselves.
- Taking care not to de-skill the supervisee.
- Insisting on the non-managerial nature of clinical supervision.

The 'skill mix' as it is sometimes called, will vary from basic listening to teaching, and perhaps advising. Any challenge will be very gentle.

Level three
- The supervisor may share his or her own experience and expertise (self-disclosure).
- Appropriate challenge will be given.
- Care will be taken not to overwhelm the supervisee with challenge.
- The non-hierarchical nature of clinical supervision may still need stressing.

Level four
- Care will be taken that the developing and deepening relationship does not result in a relaxing or blurring of boundaries.

- Referral to the contract may still be necessary.
- Avoidance of too much restorative work may be necessary.
- Mutuality is established and the supervisor encourages supervisee challenge.

Reviewing clinical supervision

You will recall that as part of the contract a recommendation that, as well as summarising each session, the whole process should be reviewed from time to time, in order to answer such questions as:

- How are we doing?
- Where are we going?
- What, if anything, needs to change?

The review would need to compare the outcomes and effectiveness of clinical supervision with the aims and objectives that were agreed at the contracting stage. The review might result in changes to the current supervision process. Such changes might include:

- Ways of working.
- The focus.
- Using a different model of supervision.

It might also, of course, cover changing the supervisor or supervisee, and this would involve a good ending (which will be covered in the final chapter). Changing the supervisor or supervisee does not need to be for negative reasons – for example, the contract may have specified a time limit, or one partner may have moved leading to practical difficulties in meeting. If an organisation was funding a supervisor, they may not wish to continue should the supervisor change employment.

Reviewing clinical supervision should have an impact on the self-awareness of supervisees, which in turn can impact on future work, both within the working alliance and within clinical practice. A small group of palliative care workers who underwent clinical supervision reviews reported that they had increased self-awareness of:

- Professional competence and limitations.
- Responses to difficulties with casework.

- Diffidence about bringing difficulties to clinical supervision and what that implied.
- Blocks (in self) to making the best use of clinical supervision.
- Feelings about responsibility and accountability.
- Feelings about the supervisor.
- Personal needs and how to address them.

The group all agreed that the review had helped them to reflect on these issues in ways they had not previously considered.

This development of self-awareness may be one of the most valuable outcomes of clinical supervision. The palliative care practitioner is constantly having to make decisions, and sometimes those decisions have to be made very quickly. This can be very stressful, and an awareness of how we came to the decision (what was I thinking then? What was I feeling? Why did I do that and not something else?) Can be a powerful way of increasing competence and so lead to more effective practice. Self-awareness can also help to answer some of the very difficult questions with which we close this chapter; try to answer them with the following definition in mind:

Palliative care is the active total care of patients whose illness no longer responds to curative treatment. It focuses on quality of life and on integrating the physical, psychological, spiritual and social aspects of care. Palliative care requires a collaborative (multi-professional) approach and follows the patient. The spectrum of palliative care provision and support required to meet patients' and carers' needs (which should be addressed throughout a patient's illness and into a carer's bereavement) ranges from the palliative care approach to specialist palliative care.

✐ Your thoughts

Is this your personal definition of palliative care? Does it reflect your personal view of what palliative care *should* be?

What has attracted you to palliative care? Why do you want to do it ? What kind of practitioner are you?

How would your colleagues describe you? How would you like your colleagues to describe you?

How would your patients/clients describe you? How would you like them to describe you?

This statement by the philosopher Aristotle from ancient Greece seems worth quoting:

> *Be what you wish to seem to be.*

If clinical supervision can move us towards this awareness, it is certainly worthwhile.

References

Hawkins P, Shohet R (1989) *Supervision in the Helping Professions.* Open University Press, Milton Keynes

Inskipp F (1998) Supervision: A Working Alliance. Alexia Publications, Sussex

CHAPTER 6

Process models

The clinical supervision models that we evaluated in *Chapter Three* were descriptions of the possible groupings for the supervision interaction(s). Remind yourself of the possibilities and re-assess your own preferences in the light of your subsequent reading.

✐ Your thoughts

What possible groupings for the supervision interactions can you think of?

As we have seen, the relationship between the supervisor and the supervisee is more complex than just two (or more) people getting together for an hour or so each month. In an attempt to capture the complexities of clinical supervision, several **process models** have been developed – some of them very complex indeed, which probably reflects how difficult it is to encapsulate the full richness of the process. In this chapter we explore some of these process models and evaluate them using some case studies.

The Six-Eyed supervisor

One of the best known models, and which is used across a range of helping professions, is the Six-Eyed supervisor. If your palliative care team has a social worker, it is very likely that this is the model with which he or she is likely to be familiar, but the model is just as suitable for other practitioners if they feel comfortable with it. The model was invented by Hawkins and Shohet (1989) and *Figure 6.1* shows an adaptation of it. It is noteworthy that it is called the Six-*Eyed* supervisor when we are exploring is super*vision*.

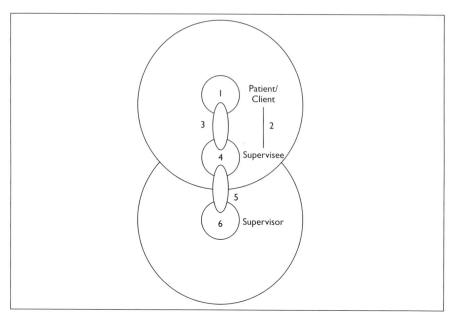

Figure 6.1: The Six-Eyed supervisor: six different ways to focus in supervision. A 'process model' adapted from Hawkins and Shohet (1989)

In the model, the numbers 1 to 6 are interpreted in the following way (try to relate each 'Eye' to the supervisee levels we looked at in *Chapter Five*).

Eye I

This eye focuses on the *content* of an interaction or intervention that the supervisee had or made with a patient or client. It will probably be mainly descriptive of what the client or patient did or said. It might include some case history to establish the context, and there is a risk that the session could then develop into a case discussion – it may not be necessary for a supervisor to know much about a patient or client. (Of course when both parties are from the same organisation, the patient may well be known to the supervisor anyway; this would also be true if colleagues were being discussed.)

✎ **Your thoughts**

How does Eye I relate to the supervisee levels in *Chapter Five?*

Eye 2

This eye represents a crucial area for clinical supervision because it is when the supervisee describes the responses, interventions, techniques and strategies they have used to help their patients or relatives. At this stage supervisees will be talking about what they did and why they did it and will be encouraged to reflect on other possible interventions. The outcomes of the interventions will be reviewed. If there is a trusting relationship, supervisees will bring not only their successes, or their 'run of the mill' work, but also work that has puzzled or distressed them and that might require some restorative work.

✐ Your thoughts

How does Eye 2 relate to the supervisee levels in *Chapter Five*?

Eye 3

The third eye is also about what happens between the supervisee and the patient or client, but it has much more to do with the dynamic of their relationship with each other. Palliative care can sometimes have an image that was once expressed to me as: 'it gets on my nerves – everything is supposed to be so perfect – angels singing and violins playing – ugh! What actually happens is a lot more down to earth let me tell you!'. In the intimacy of palliative care the nature of the relationship between practitioner (the supervisee) and patient can be very profound, but it is a mistake to assume that this means that the relationship will therefore be *easy*. In any relationship, those involved will have feelings about each other – it would be rather worrying if this were not so! – But to assume that those feelings will invariably be positive is not realistic. A practitioner will always try to be professional, of course, but inevitably some personal feelings will exist (similarly for the patient or client). For example, if the dying person is very angry, that anger may get directed at the practitioner. But *liking* an angry person isn't easy, even when we understand the reasons for the anger and feel compassion. The third 'Eye' aims to look at how a supervisee interprets the dynamic – what is going on between the two? What happens at beginnings and endings? Who or what does the patient (or the patient's relatives) see the helper *as*?.

✐ Your thoughts

How does Eye 3 relate to the supervisee levels in *Chapter Five?*

Eye 4

The focus here is on the internal processes of the supervisee. The supervisor will encourage exploration of personal thoughts and feelings, especially those that may not have been congruent with what they were *doing* with or for a patient or client. For example: while efficiently setting up a syringe driver, a nurse at the end of a tiring day might be thinking how good it will be to get home, and might be hoping that a relative won't want to talk and cause a delay. The supervisor, in a non-judgemental way may encourage ventilation of the feelings to help the practitioner consider issues about workload, or about the choice between becoming 'too involved' (always a strong injunction for all care practitioners) and becoming 'distant'. No doubt you can think of other examples of how it might be quite illuminating to explore feelings about clients and patients.

✐ Your thoughts

How does Eye 4 relate to the supervisee levels in *Chapter Five?*

Eye 5

We have emphasised the importance of the working alliance relationship between the supervisor and supervisee; the fifth Eye requires the focus to be on the dynamic between the two. What is actually going on between them right now? There is a theory called **parallel process** (which we look at in greater detail later) that suggests that what is going on in the dynamic between the patient, client or colleague and the supervisee will be reflected in the dynamic of the supervisory relationship. We have mentioned that problems can arise in the supervisory relationship (for example there may be competitiveness) and it might be worth trying to establish whether there is some sort of power issue with the patient (eg 'they just never do as I ask – even though it's to help them') which is showing up in clinical supervision in a different form.

📎 **Your thoughts**

How does Eye 5 relate to the supervisee levels in *Chapter Five?*

Eye 6

Finally, the supervisor needs to examine his or her own processes, just as the supervisee does in Eye 4. The supervisor will be trying to be aware of what is happening in the 'here and now' of the working alliance. Questions that come to mind are:

- What do I think I am doing here?
- Am I really helping my supervisee?
- Am I really helping the patients/clients?
- Do I have any doubts? (About practice? About my competence?)
- Where are we going with this?

📎 **Your thoughts**

How does Eye 6 relate to the supervisee levels in *Chapter Five?*

Re-read each of the six 'Eyes' and try to fix the model in your mind. Then read the following case study and try to note where any of the 'Eyes' might be operating.

👁 **Witness statement**

Mary is a hospice home-care nurse. Clinical supervision is relatively new for her and she is very enthusiastic about it.

Mary I want to talk to you about Brian. You know, the young man with all those awkward relatives that we discussed last time.

Clinical supervisor Mmmmm.

Mary The doctor has increased the medication and that's okay, I know what I'm doing, but it's Brian – he keeps asking me whether the medication is killing him and wants me to tackle Dr John. He can get quite aggressive, accusing me, well us... I suppose, of trying to speed up his death.

Clinical supervisor Tell me what you say when he asks.

Mary Well – that's just it. I don't know what to say. It's pointless getting into an argument with him, but I can't just ignore it can I?

Clinical supervisor So what *do* you do?

Mary Yes, hmm. Well...I suppose I just change the subject.

Clinical supervisor And does that work?

Mary Not really, I suppose, because he just comes back to it. It's hard, because although he's never been the easiest of patients, I've grown quite fond of him and now I think he probably doesn't trust me and I've worked really hard to gain his trust.

Clinical supervisor And that's rather hurtful?

Mary Yes, it is to be honest. But I'm stuck – I seem to be caught between the devil and ...

Clinical supervisor What might being honest achieve?

Mary You mean telling him that the medication is to ease his pain, but that it could have other effects too?

Clinical supervisor Mmm. But I was thinking more about sharing your own feelings with him.

✎ **Your thoughts**

Can you see where any of the six 'Eyes' might be operating?

I expect you noted something of 'Eyes' 1, 2, 3, 4 and 6.

1. Mary first describes Brian and the problem
2. Mary describes her reactions and what she did and didn't do.
3. Mary is gently encouraged to look at her relationship with Brian.
4. Challenge about congruence is introduced (What might being honest achieve?').
5. The supervisor self-discloses ('...I was thinking...').

A question you may have pondered on is how or whether the participants could be aware of all these 'eyes' as the clinical supervision session proceeds. With practice it is possible, but record taking (which we look at in the next chapter) is a good way of re-visiting a session in order to examine the process as well as the content. In the case study, recording the session actually threw up some issues relevant to Eye 5, as it became clear that what mary was really wanting her supervisor to do was to tell her what to do, because she still regarded him as a sort of manager or consultant.

The clinical rhombus model

In this model the supervisor is placed at the peak of the figure because, in the supervisory role, *all* the relationships of the key players need to be kept in view. For instance, the relationship between practitioner (P) and client/patient (C/P) and between practitioner (supervisee) (P) and supervisor (CS) are clearly very important. However, the supervisor may have been appointed by an agency or by the organisation and may be bound by a code of practice, with an equal responsibility to the patient(s) or client(s). Perceived practitioner 'not good enough' practice cannot continue at the expense of the welfare of service users. It may be very painful to intervene on a service user's behalf, but supervisors have to carry that responsibility, and therefore need to be aware of the relationships involved – hence the link from CS↔C/P in the diagram. The fourth corner of the model (A) is seen as the hospital, clinic, or hospice which provided the clinical supervision (and maybe paid for it) and which refers patients to the practitioner. The supervisor therefore has a relationship with this a corner and so does the practitioner, and in both cases the relationship may be quite complex and sometimes conflicting because financial, organisational and ethical aspects might be present.

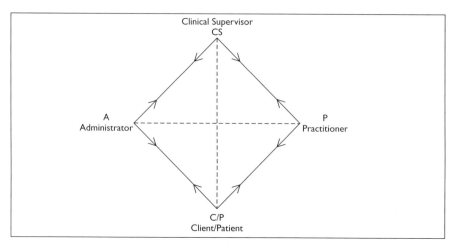

Figure 6.2: The clinical rhombus model

The inventors of the model, Eckstein and Wallerstein (1978), suggest that the model can work in both content and process ways:

The practitioner has to work to help the patient and to do this needs knowledge and skills to cope with the work (P↔C/P). The supervisor will work to meet these needs and the material brought by the supervisee will foster learning and competence (P↔CS) The A figure will affect these tasks. Thus far, the model would be fulfilling the formative and normative functions of clinical supervision (inasmuch as it is more content than process).

In process terms, the supervisee's relationship with the patient (P↔C/P) requires more than skill and knowledge, because the practitioner's own self is involved and just 'applying' skills and knowledge will not be sufficient. In the therapeutic use of self, formative and normative interventions alone would probably be inadequate.

The supervisor (CS) is not the supervisee's counsellor or therapist, but in order to help the clinical work with the patient, and to increase and develop the supervisee's competence, some work on the dynamics of the supervisee's relationship with the patient (CS↔P) will be needed and this is likely to mean at least some exploration of the supervisee's own feelings. This would perhaps come under the restorative function.

While the A figure may in content terms represent the requirements within which both parties work, it may also represent many other aspects of work – frustration, resentment, suspicion and a host of other negatives, as well as (we might hope) some positive ones.

Below is a case study that illustrates the clinical rhombus model in practice (as you read, refer to the diagram above and then evaluate the model for your own practice).

☞ The clinical rhombus model in practice

The supervisor (CS) is employed by a hospice to supervise the work of the social worker who also runs the bereavement service. She is newly trained as a counsellor in addition to her social work qualification and takes bereavement clients who may be thought too difficult for the bereavement volunteers. The supervisor is paid by the hospice, but is not required to give any account of the work, except to record when and where it took place. Externally, the rhombus looks like the one illustrated in *Figure 6.3*.

The flow along the lines can be quite complex: with the (A) corner having considerable power: it pays the supervisor, it pays the social worker's salary, and expects a high standard of work on a very heavy caseload, which it is the agent for providing. It also provides the setting in which the clinical supervision and much of the social worker's activity takes place.

The social worker needs to be sure that although the (A) figure funds the clinical supervision, the supervisor is not therefore in a line-management position. The social worker has little choice in the matter of patients and clients and is expected to pick up all referrals. The supervisor has a responsibility to deliver quality work (especially as she knows that hospice funds are always 'stretched'). She is aware that there are problems on the Practitioner↔Administrator line (P↔A), particularly to do with a sense of being punished for her success by being overloaded with cases.

The process work revolved around the practitioner's difficulty in working as a counsellor with some clients, particularly those on medication. She brought this to supervision as a point for fairly abstract discussion: 'does medication interfere with grief?'. Working with the supervisee's feelings about the medicated clients, the supervisor was able to establish that the difficulties had much more to do with frustration that there was no choice in the matter of referrals. The difficulties were actually to do with the system (the A figure).

Additionally, because the supervisee was new to counselling, she tended to want the supervisor to tell her what to do and this was awkward for the supervisor, who did not see this as her role, who was concerned not to de-skill the supervisee, and who was also anxious that telling someone what to do or not do could result in the same thing happening with clients and patients ('my supervisor said you/I should —'). The supervisor was also aware of her own feelings about being overloaded and did not wish to over-sympathise.

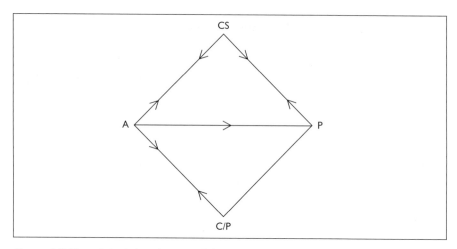

Figure 6.3: The clinical rhombus model in practice

Parallel Process

It is from the clinical rhombus model that the concept of **parallel process** developed (although it was first mentioned by Searles (1955), which is now accepted as an element of virtually all process models. The model has been described (Searles, 1955) as:

> *The processes at work currently in the relationship between client and worker are often reflected in the relationship between worker and supervisor.*

The idea is that although supervisees will attempt to convey their material accurately, some aspects of their work will have involved material that has conveyed itself at a deeper, less conscious level. This transmission is thought to occur more frequently with 'difficult' or 'disturbed' patients. For instance, a normally clear and articulate supervisee may become muddled or confused and the supervisor would explore whether the patient was also muddled or confused, or how the client was affecting the supervisee. To work effectively with parallel process a supervisor needs to be very alert to and aware of his or her own thoughts, feelings and imaginings, and even the physical sensations aroused by the supervisee's material. (This may remind you of the Eye 6). Reactions can then be relayed to the supervisee to enable greater insight into the patient–practitioner relationship (PC↔P). Consider this example of how the supervisor's reactions were offered to a practitioner:

As you can see, the process can work in more than one way, and may result from the supervisee's work or from the supervisor's feelings.

It is worth mentioning that some very eminent writers, including Feltham and Dryden (1994). have serious reservations about parallel process. It is pointed out that parallel process is not a *fact*, but a name attached to an experience, or even to an intuition, that has manifested itself in clinical supervision for some people. The reservations are that some supervisors do regard it as a fact and so tend to watch for it and point it out, almost as if it *must* be present.

What do you see as the dangers here?

Care needs to be taken that the supervisor's 'ah-ha!' sense of the presence of parallel process really does match up with the material presented by the supervisee. Also, a good enough relationship needs to exist for a supervisee to be able to challenge whether the supervisor is accurate. One way of checking is to monitor any differences in reaction(s): for instance the supervisor might notice that sessions with some supervisees pass very, very quickly, yet once in a while a session seems to drag. The supervisor might check whether this is also happening in the practitioner–client/patient sessions (P↔CP), but would not automatically assume that parallel process is present.

Pointing out parallel process indiscriminately could well de-skill a supervisee, who might worry that they had overlooked it. Other negatives could be that the supervisee becomes self-conscious (as opposed to self-aware) with the patient or client. It could also result in material being 'doctored' before presentation, if the supervisee thinks that the supervisor will be scrutinising every interaction for parallel process.

The bi-lateral process model

You may have heard of or have experience of transactional analysis (TA). It is a theory of personality which has gained popularity not only in counselling and therapy arenas, but also in business and organisations and for teams. The theory proposes that we all interact (TA uses the term 'transact' – we make 'transactions' with each other) from three ego states as shown in *Figure 6.4*.

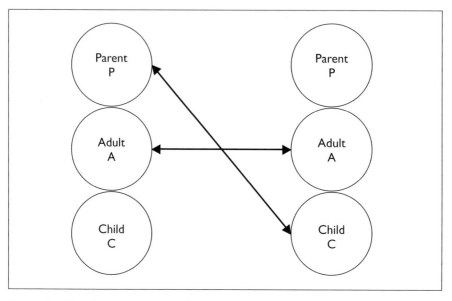

Figure 6.4:The three ego states of transactional analysis

You can see that there can be a variety of transactions. Remember that Parent, Adult, Child does not refer to actual parents, adults, and children, but to the ways in which we respond from those parts of ourselves, thus:

- Adult↔Adult might be a practitioner asking a patient 'How are you today?' and a response from the patient 'Not too bad. About the same as yesterday.'
- Adult↔Child might be 'How are you today?' with the response 'Lousy, and I don't know why you ask. As if you care!'

Apply this to some transactions from your own experience.

✎ **Your thoughts**

Can you think of any examples of transactions from your own experience:
- Adult↔Adult?
- Adult↔Child?

Okay-ness

Another popular idea in transactional analysis is the notion of 'okay-ness' as shown in *Figure 6.5*.

1 I'm OK You're OK	2 I'm OK You're not OK
4 I'm not OK You're not OK	3 I'm not OK You're OK

Figure 6.5: Okay-ness

You might find it fun to list where you think you, your colleagues, your patients, their relatives operate from on the grid (make sure that any people you use are made anonymous):

Can you apply the 'okay-ness' grid:
- To yourself?
- To colleagues?
- To patients and clients?
- To relatives of patients?

Game playing

The third idea in transactional analysis involves 'games'. These games are psychological transactions that we have learned through life, which we use as a defence, to blame others or as a way of manipulating others, or – worst of all – as a way of undermining or attacking others. Berne, the originator of transactional analysis (Berne, 1968, 1972) gave names to these games, but they can easily be recognised from the ways in which they are introduced (for example 'If it weren't for you/my spouse/my parents/ my teachers...'). This game is called 'wooden leg' ('If it weren't for my wooden leg, I could run in the Olympics') and it is used as an excuse for not taking responsibility.

Clinical supervision is not immune from game-playing and we'll look at some of the games played in supervision sessions later. A process model for clinical supervision has been devised by two specialists in the field of transactional analysis.

As you can see this process is very complex, but it does have the advantage of attempting to envisage the position of both parties. Try to put yourself in the position of A and then of B. Then check whether the models? Are present in this transcription of part of a clinical supervision session between a specialist palliative care nurse and her supervisor. They have worked together for some time and have mutual respect and trust.

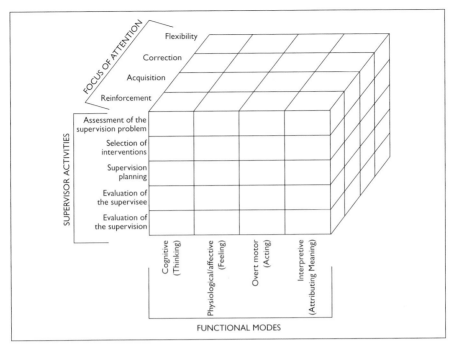

Figure 6.6: Practitioner operations in the supervisory process

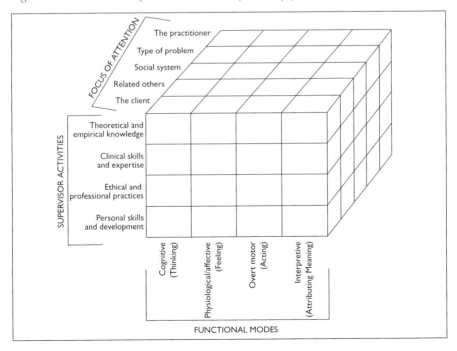

Figure 6.7: Supervisor operations in the supervisory process

👁 **Witness statement**

Nurse I have a real problem with this patient. She really gets to me. She's always sort of critical and ungrateful – not that I want patients to be grateful, but she's *always* dissatisfied and somehow disapproving.

Clinical supervisor OK, that's her. Tell me a bit about how you work with her. What skills do you use?

Nurse Well, other than the practical stuff (which is easy) I keep trying to be pleasant and courteous. I mean, I hope I'm always professional, it wouldn't, like, be ethical to be anything else, would it?

Clinical supervisor I'm not clear what exactly the problem is. You seem to be operating OK.

Nurse I just don't like her and that bothers me. It's never happened to me before, even with quite difficult people. I can't fathom it.

Clinical supervisor You think you should like your patients, as well as respect them, perhaps?

Nurse I suppose not, but it does help!

Clinical supervisor Tell me how others in the team find her.

Nurse I don't know, I've never asked. [with a wry grin] I guess I worry in case *they* like her!

Clinical supervisor So maybe you feel the problem is more you than the patient? Sort of your beliefs and values.

Jot down how you felt about this model.

✎ **Your thoughts**

What do you think about the supervisor and practitioner models in this transaction?

It is difficult, I think you'll agree, to check what aspects are evidenced here, and some would certainly be realised only in a retrospective reflective view of the session, rather than being experienced in the session itself. Some people who use this model have copies of it and at the end of each session take a few minutes to colour in the blocks or squares which seem to have been present until, over time, they agree and can feel satisfied that all have been covered.

The Practice-centred model

Finally, here is a process model which is partly functional and partly process. It was trialled in thirty NHS trusts. It is called a practice-centred model (Nicklin, 1997) and is illustrated as shown in *Figure 6.8*.

It is a far less complex than the models we have reviewed so far, and

Managerial
Clinical standards;
Clinical procedures;
Employment policies:
appraisal, discipline,
grievance;
Case work analysis;
Workload management.

Educational
Statutory education;
In-service training;
Mentorship;
Preceptorship;
Personal development;
Planning;
Research.

Supportive
Personal services;
Welfare services;
Occupational health;
Peer support;
Counselling.

practice
analysis

evaluation

problem
identification

implementation
action

objective
setting

planning

Figure 6.8: The practice-centred model: Practice analysis: *the practitioner's problem situation/s is/are explored. Examination of a specific situation (examplar), case history, or incident (critical incident analysis) may be helpful in illuminating concerns about clinical competence, workload management, relationships with colleagues and clients, and personal and professional development.* Problem identification: *is closely related to practice analysis, but moves from exploration to clarification. Problems are frequently expressed in vague terms and the problem has to be stated specifically, but not before the objective of the proposed actions is clearly understood.* Objective setting: *too often this stage of the problem-solving cycle receives scant attention or is ignored entirely. Objectives framed in the context of practice seek to confirm the expectations, obligations and aspirations of the organisation, patient, the profession, and the individual practitioner. It is at this stage that discrepancies and perverse consequences of subsequent action will be identified.* Planning: *is concerned with agreeing specific and realistic action within an agreed time-frame using available resources. Selecting options may be aided by techniques such as force-field analysis. 'Doing nothing' is always an option, but only if it is selected as such, and not merely the failure to take agreed action.* Implementation and action: *the practitioner implements the agreed action. The supervisor may, of course, act as a resource or may have access to information or resources, but responsibility for problems, objectives and action is with the practitioner.* Evaluation: *is of two types – evaluation of the outcomes of supervision (the agreed action) and of the supervision process itself*

this may lend it appeal. Its practical, down-to-earth approach contrasts (perhaps for some practitioners, favourably) with the bi-lateral model and it is easily linked to formative, normative and restorative functions of clinical supervision. It has a solution-focused action base and this may further add to its appeal. Palliative care is, however, a very complex area of work and the other models may feel more appropriate for the complexity of the work and the personal challenges it presents.

In your evaluation of the model, you might reflect on whether it offers more or less than other models.

Other models

Illustrations of two further process models are given in the addendum at the end of the chapter and you might like to explore these for yourself. They are:
■ The double helix model
■ A systems model (which includes organisational factors).

In conclusion

This chapter has attempted to cover some fairly complex material. Process models do not make the easiest of reading! Exploring process, whether in clinical supervision or in any other discipline (group process is a prime example) demands a high level of concentration and, in contrast to exploring content, can be quite demanding. Yet this is – in a sense – its purpose.

Palliative care work *is* demanding – it demands high levels of skill, commitment, stamina, patience, compassion and a host of other attributes. This is the precise reason for our need to reflect on our work and to become aware of its complexity at many levels, so that we can ensure that it is not just 'good enough' but that it exemplifies excellence. Practitioners who only 'do their job' (even if they do it well) are unlikely to be personally challenged and they are unlikely to be challenging themselves. If we do not take the time and apply some energy to asking ourselves certain questions our development both as practitioners and as people will be stunted. Such questions might include:

■ What was I doing then?

- Why was I doing it?
- Did I have a choice?
- How did I make that choice?
- Why did I make the choice I did?

We may well be 'good enough' but is that good enough? Elizabeth Kübler-Ross, to whom palliative care owes so much, said (Kübler-Ross, 1988):

> *All the trials and tribulations, and the biggest losses that you ever experience, things that make you say 'If I had known about this I would never have been able to make it through' are gifts for you. It's like somebody had to – what do you call that when you make the hot iron into a tool? – you have to temper the tool. It is an opportunity that you are given to grow. That is the sole purpose of existence on this planet Earth. You will not grow if you sit in a beautiful flower garden and somebody brings you gorgeous food on a silver platter. But you will grow if you are sick, if you experience losses and if you do not put your head in the sand, but take the pain and learn to accept it, not as a curse or a punishment, but as a gift to you with a very, very specific purpose.*

She was, of course, writing about pain and loss, but her words could well be applied to what good clinical supervision can do for us and for our practice, and ultimately for palliative care itself.

References

Berne E(1968) *Games People Play*. Grove Press, New York

Berne E (1972) *What Do You Say After You Say 'Hello'?*. Corgi Books, London

Eckstein R, Wallerstein RW (1978) *The Teaching and Learning of Psychotherapy*. International Universities Press, New York

Feltham C, Dryden W (1994) *Developing Counsellor Supervision* Sage Publications, London

Hawkins P, Shohet R (1989) *Supervision in the Helping Professions*. Open University Press, Milton Keynes

Kübler-Ross E (1969) *On Death and Dying*. Touchstone, New York

Mattinson J (1975) *The Reflection Process in Case Work Supervision*.

Institute of Marital Studies, London

Nicklin P (1997) A practice centred model of clinical supervision. *Nursing Times* **93**(46)

Searles HF (1955) The informational value of the supervisor's emotional experience. in: *Collected Papers on Schizophrenia and Related Subjects.* Hogarth Press, London

Van Ooijen E (2000) *Clinical Supervision: A Practical Guide.* Churchill Livingstone, Edinburgh

Addendum to Chapter Six

The double-helix model of supervision

This model shows the integration between the structure, process and outcome double helices.

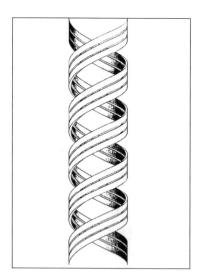

The Holloway model of supervision

This is adapted from Holloway E (1995) The systems model of supervision in clinical supervision. In: Holloway E. *A Systems Approach to Supervision.* Sage Publications, London.

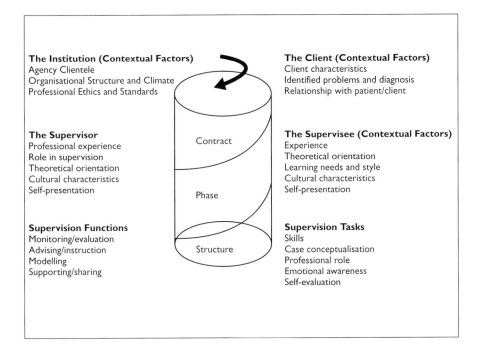

The Institution (Contextual Factors)
Agency Clientele
Organisational Structure and Climate
Professional Ethics and Standards

The Supervisor
Professional experience
Role in supervision
Theoretical orientation
Cultural characteristics
Self-presentation

Supervision Functions
Monitoring/evaluation
Advising/instruction
Modelling
Supporting/sharing

Contract

Phase

Structure

The Client (Contextual Factors)
Client characteristics
Identified problems and diagnosis
Relationship with patient/client

The Supervisee (Contextual Factors)
Experience
Theoretical orientation
Learning needs and style
Cultural characteristics
Self-presentation

Supervision Tasks
Skills
Case conceptualisation
Professional role
Emotional awareness
Self-evaluation

CHAPTER 7

Record taking, record keeping and other ethical matters

The business of records – taking them, keeping them, destroying them – can often be a major issue in clinical supervision (as we saw in *Chapter Four*), although it need not be. The issue often creates embarrassment at the contracting stage and many supervisees report it as an on-going chore.

What are your views?

✏ Your thoughts

Are you for or against record taking and record keeping? What are your reasons?

List your reasons for:
List your reasons against:

At a most basic level it is obvious that if an organisation is giving time (or time off in lieu) or is paying in other ways for clinical supervision then it will quite reasonably want to know that meetings have taken place. A simple record would at least show that participants had met regularly and this would provide evidence for some sort of audit of the benefits of clinical supervision. Few people have any problem with this. The information might, however, be more useful if the issues discussed in the sessions were bullet-pointed, particularly if the content of the discussion might lead to improvements in service care. The shaded box shows what a supervisor and supervisee said about records when they were interviewed for this book.

◉ Witness statement

Supervisee (a palliative care nurse) Initially I was a bit nervous about records. It all seemed too formal –a bit over the top.
Clinical supervisor I was nervous about discussing it, because I thought it might put her off (I was new to clinical supervision then) but in my training I'd been convinced that it was crucial, so I ploughed on!
Supervisee In the end, it was quite easy. We printed off a form, with our names and spaces for dates and times and then left five or ten minutes at the end of each session listing the topics we'd worked on, but not what we'd said about the topics. And we each signed a copy.
Clinical supervisor Yes, I remember that a recurrent topic was THE CAR PARK! But the great thing about our system was that it took some pressure off where the notes should be kept and who had access, because they didn't mean anything to anyone else.
Supervisee I was won over because I can add the record form to my portfolio for PREP.

This nurse had a sound practical reason for keeping records, but suspicion about record keeping can often be dispelled by focusing on the fact that records can evidence success!

Here is an example of a form used in a hospice, which seems very like the one devised by the two interviewees. It can be easily printed and used as a pro forma by everyone engaged in clinical supervision. It has the advantage of being brief and of being impersonal, because it lists topics and issues, but not people or personalities.

☞ Example of a record of clinical supervision

Name of supervisor:_____

Name of supervisee(s):_____

Length of session met for: _____

Date of meeting: _____

Items covered during session: _____

We both/we all agree with this record. _____

Supervisor's signature: _____

Supervisee(s) signature(s):_____

Reasons for record taking

It is easy to assume that we will carry full and clear memories in our heads of what happened in each supervision session (also remember that a supervisor may have more than one supervisee). A few (very few) people might indeed be able to do this. But for most of us it will not be possible and in the busy world of palliative care memories of what was said a month ago may get a bit blurred around the edges, to say the least. It is also interesting that what is remembered vividly by one party may not have had the same significance for the other party. This can sometimes lead to hurt feelings that could potentially damage the relationship, as the following statement from a bereavement visitor shows:

👁 Witness statement

We'd had a very good session and I went off full of ideas about how to work with a family I'd been feeling rather stuck with. I was bursting to tell [the supervisor] how it had all gone, but she looked rather blank as if she didn't really know what I was talking about. I felt a bit 'flat' to tell you the truth.

Do you think a record would have helped here? In what way?

✏ Your thoughts

How would record keeping have helped here?

A further advantage is that records can save time: had there been even a brief record of this session, the supervisor could have reminded herself of what had transpired in the previous session, and this would have avoided repetition of the material and ensured continuity, as well as avoiding hurt feelings.

We could also envisage a 'worst-case scenario' where a practitioner is involved in some kind of disciplinary hearing. The fact that he or she had been receiving regular clinical supervision could have a significant bearing on the outcome. I hope that you will never be involved in this kind of unhappy situation, but the following true story may serve to illustrate how important records can be.

Case report

Catherine was a palliative care nurse attached to an oncology department. She had serious misgivings about the way in which her colleagues, instructed by senior colleagues, were interpreting the Kübler-Ross model of dying, which consists of the following stages:

- denial
- anger
- bargaining
- depression
- acceptance.

She thought that following the stages so rigidly was not necessarily the same as 'following' the patient and his or her illness. She was especially uncomfortable with the sense, as she put it, that 'You had to get them through to acceptance or else you'd failed'. She also thought that the evidence of her own eyes showed that the model was not true for all patients, all of the time, and that there was some inaccurate interpretation of Kübler-Ross's model anyway.

Eventually she began to sense that she was increasingly unpopular with some of her colleagues. A grievance was taken up against her. It was expressed in a variety of ways that she was practising in a way detrimental to patients' well-being. Really she felt that it was her refusal to follow the preferred model rigidly. She had voiced her unhappiness several times in clinical supervision, and records showing this were available to demonstrate that she was a thoughtful and reflective practitioner and that her concerns were not trivial, but showed a real concern for patient welfare. The disciplinary panel dismissed the grievance.

Take a moment to jot down your thoughts about Catherine's predicament.

✐ Your thoughts

What do you think about this practitioner's interpretation of the Kübler-Ross model?

Extensive note taking can be very tedious, and then it becomes difficult to sustain the discipline. At the contract-making stage it is probably essential to make a decision about two things as far as record taking is concerned:

- Is the supervisee expected to bring notes about his or her practice to the clinical supervision sessions? If so – what form should they take?
- Will both parties make records of the actual sessions? If so, when and how will they be made?

A supervisor and supervisee were interviewed separately on this issue. What follows is what they said about records.

◉ Witness statement

Clinical supervisor I find it really helpful if they bring a list with them of what they want to discuss. It needn't be that long, but it makes better use of the time if we don't have to have a long narrative about what they've been doing. I find that it helps me to focus and seems to give a structure to the session.

Supervisee (a hospice social worker) It's a bit of a chore, but I'm always glad when I get there that I've got some notes. It's so easy to get anecdotal, and then before you know it the time's gone and you haven't got to what you really needed help with. I always try to give the list a sort of order of priority too, just in case we run out of time.

Methods of record taking

If as a supervisor you agree with the supervisee that notes will be brought to the sessions, you will want to devise a system that is not too time-consuming or onerous. The easier the system is the more likely it is that recording will take place and that the records will be useful, and that looking at them will not take up too much of the actual session time. Jot down what information you, as a supervisor, would find helpful.

Your supervisee may well be accustomed to taking case notes, but this is not really what is required for clinical supervision. Case notes (quite rightly) keep the focus on the patient or client – the notes for clinical supervision should be on the supervisee's work *with* the patient or client (a point we have tried to emphasise about the focus of supervision throughout this text).

Two well-known methods of recording are illustrated in *Figures 7.1* and *7.2.* You may well be familiar with these methods because they are often used to encourage reflective practice. But they are equally useful for

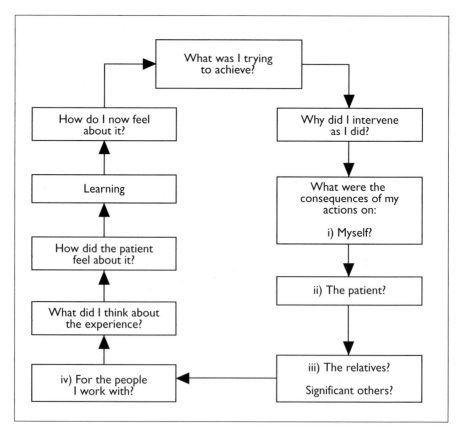

Figure 7.1: Model of structured reflection

preparing for clinical supervision – or a supervisor could use the questions to guide the supervisee. If all the *I's* in the Gibbs model, for instance, are turned into *you's* there would be excellent focus on supervisee work with patients or clients. The focus should also help make best use of time.

A very similar model is included in the addendum to this chapter.

A great advantage of these methods is that they can also be used to structure the supervision session. Take a typical incident that you would like to discuss or analyse and use the two methods to help you structure the incident and your interventions, as if you were preparing for clinical supervision.

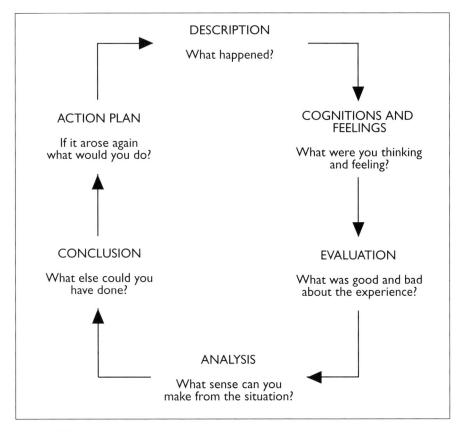

Figure 7.2: The reflective cycle

✏ **Your thoughts**

Can you give structure to your typical incident and interventions using both methods of recording?

- Structured reflection
- Reflective cycle

A useful spin-off for nurses is that these records could be used as portfolio evidence, just as suggested by the nurse quoted earlier. (Some further methods of recording are given in the addendum at the end of the chapter.)

Storage of records

The conversation above about note-taking revealed concern about where any records might be kept. If they contain sensitive or controversial material, their security is important. In the world of palliative care, security may have particular significance, because it is a relatively small world, where people (whether patients or colleagues) may be readily identified. In an average-sized hospice, for example, if clinical supervision is provided internally then it is highly likely that a supervisor will recognise people who are discussed as part of the supervisory work, even if they were made anonymous. Indeed the people may already have been discussed at a case meeting where both parties were present.

This highlights the importance of the *content* of the notes or records and, if they are to be seen by others, the security of where and how they are stored. Collecting paper and storing it, often, it would seem, for the sake of it, is one of the besetting problems of current times; clinical supervision should not exacerbate the problem. So a decision to keep notes and records to a minimum and to keep them discreet is in itself very sensible, but retaining them and deciding who shall have access to them may present a few obstacles. In the electronic age it is possible to store records on a computer, but security is equally important here, and what if the system crashes? Would it matter? The Access to Information Act (2000) and the Data Protection Act (1998) may seem a little 'over the top' for a few simple notes jotted down at the end of a clinical supervision hour, but some of the points they make about data protection may be useful to think about as a guide. The Freedom of Information Act (2000) may also need to be considered.

- The Data Protection Act (1998) gives people the right to access information about them held on computers, and in some instances to handwritten records.
- Records must be protected against misuse. This means that it's important to know who will have access and that those individuals will not misuse the information. Someone who should not have access could possibly misuse information, even accidentally, so it is as well to take care.
- Records must be kept only for a specific purpose, so think carefully about having a valid reason for storing them, should you be challenged.
- Records must be accurate and 'relevant to the matter in hand'.
- Records must be up to date and should not be kept beyond the point where they might be seen as irrelevant or unnecessary. But this is a very tricky point. How is it possible to decide whether what you discussed in clinical supervision last month will be relevant next year? If the records are kept for a PREP (Post-Registration Education and Practice) portfolio, or for presentation at a future job interview, then how long into the future should that be?

All of this may make you think 'Why bother?'. Make a list of why it is worthwhile to 'bother'.

✐ Your thoughts

Why we should bother with record keeping?

Here are some of the positive reasons for record keeping, which were contributed by a variety of palliative care workers.

👁 Witness statements

They have been useful for refreshing my memory. My days are so full and I seem to see so many people in between sessions that I'd never remember what to talk about if I didn't write it down.

cont../.

The records give me a real opportunity to reflect on my practice when I look back over them at a later date.

Sometimes we set goals (mainly for me, but sometimes for both of us in terms of where we are with the supervision) and the records are a good way of monitoring how the goals are progressing. Am I getting there?

The notes help me to see whether any changes have taken place – either with me or with the clients.

My supervisor moved away and it was very good to look at what we'd achieved before we ended.

I was very glad of the records when several of us needed to show that we'd tried really hard to resolve a rather nasty issue.

In our hospice the same issue kept on raising its head time after time. Our clinical supervision records helped to provide statistical evidence without having to name names.

We wanted to make a case for keeping clinical supervision after the trial period ended and the records meant that we could show the benefits.

✐ Your thoughts

Where will your notes and records be kept (at home? at work? on a computer? in a filing cabinet?).

Who would you or wouldn't you want to have access to your notes?

What might you think or feel if you were asked to produce your notes as 'evidence' (of meetings, of interventions, of good or poor practice by self or others)?

Look back at the models described in *Chapter Two*. How would the keeping of records and their security affect group or network supervision?

Ethics of record keeping

Records and their security is an ethical issue. What does the term 'ethical' mean to you/for you?

✎ **Your thoughts**

What does the term 'ethical' mean to you?

At its most basic level, the word 'ethics' relates to the study of right and wrong behaviour. And in palliative care it has special significance because of the nature of the work which quite literally is a 'life and death' matter and because of the vulnerability of the patients, clients, and those near to them. Working ethically may mean adherence to a particular code of ethics and code of practice: in a palliative care team, as we mentioned earlier, different colleagues may adhere to different codes. A hospice usually has a large cohort of volunteers who may or may not be bound by a code, but who nevertheless work ethically. You will remember that in *Chapter One* you were asked for your view of the following statement by a well-known writer on supervision (Carroll, 1996):

> *Ethical codes do not give answers to many individual situations, and it is here that clinical supervision can provide a forum that alerts to ethical sensitivity and allows for reflection preceding decisions.*

Carroll seems to indicate that adherence to a code is not sufficient for the individual concerns or problems which crop up day by day in the field of care. Think of an ethical issue, problem or concern that you have encountered. If you subscribe to or know of a code, try to decide whether reference to it would have helped when you tried to resolve it. Would it have helped to discuss it with another professional? In what way?

✎ **Your thoughts**

How would you use a code you are familiar with too resolve an ethical problem?

- Issue or problem
- Code used
- Level of help it offered
- Further help needed (if any)

Remind yourself of the formative, normative, restorative and perspective functions of clinical supervision. Which do you think would be covered by a code?

✐ **Your thoughts**

Which of the functions of clinical supervision are likely to be covered by a code?

- Formative?
- Normative?
- Restorative?
- Perspective?

Codes are unlikely to cover the restorative function, and yet being able to share concerns and anxieties about ethical issues may be the first step towards solving any problems and lead to greater clarity. Records and their security (which we have discussed) are closely linked to confidentiality, and confidentiality is certainly an ethical matter, and being clear about the boundaries of confidentiality is essential for ethical practice.

Make a list of what you regard as confidential:

✐ **Your thoughts**

What information would it be okay to disclose?
What information would you not disclose?
What information are you a bit uncertain about disclosing?

Then decide how you could present these boundaries in your clinical supervision contract.

Responsibility in record keeping

Earlier in the book we discussed **responsibility** in some depth. Awareness of our responsibilities to and for our patients, clients, colleagues, organisations and ourselves is also an ethical issue. Remind yourself of the responsibilities you identified for yourself as supervisor and supervisee in *Chapter Two*. Would you say that responsibility is an ethical issue?

✐ **Your thoughts**

Do you agree or disagree that responsibility is an ethical issue? What are your reasons?

A further ethical consideration concerns working within one's own level of competence. A supervisor will be alert to signs that a practitioner is out of his or her depth and will try to remedy the situation by suggesting additional training, some personal counselling, or other appropriate help. It is also important that supervisors are equally aware of their own levels of competence as supervisors, and take steps to update or improve their practice.

Ending of the working alliance

Sometimes limits of competence may mean that the working alliance will come to an end, and there may be other reasons for bringing a supervisory relationship to an end. Endings have a particular poignancy in palliative care, as they so often mean the closure of a life as well as of a relationship. Bringing a supervisory relationship to a satisfactory end is therefore not only important in itself, but also has ethical implications, as we should be modelling the 'good' endings we strive to have with patients and clients. Endings should be planned, structured, and even contracted if they are to be successful. There should be a mutually agreed timing and process for bringing the relationship to an end. This will involve:

1. Providing opportunities for the supervisee to acknowledge change(s) in practice, and progress towards the original or revised outcomes and goals. Issues worked through during the working alliance can be reviewed, as can professional development and any successes or failures. The supervisee might also want to reflect on met and unmet needs – not as a criticism of the supervisor, but in terms of on-going professional development.

2. Using the boundaries of the supervisory relationship to assist the ending. This could involve working through or reducing dependency, if the supervisee seems concerned about self-reliance. It might mean re-asserting or modelling the nature of the contract and re-visiting what was agreed about the nature of the working alliance.

The supervisor can make a significant contribution to the ending by:

- 'letting go' in a positive and clear manner
- by acknowledging feelings of loss
- by encouraging reflection on work achieved and its implications for patients and clients
- by offering to help with future arrangements for clinical supervision
- by affirming the Supervisee's autonomy.

There should be an opportunity to discuss any unresolved issues and to decide what should happen about these.

Try to list your own feelings about endings.

✐ Your thoughts

What are your feelings about endings?

Just as it is difficult to give absolute guidance as to how long records should be kept, it is not easy to give firm 'rules' about when a particular working alliance should draw to a close. If both/all parties feel that they are working productively and if there is sound evidence that their work is benefiting clients and patients then it may seem pointless and wasteful to terminate it. On the other hand, no single supervisor can be all things to all supervisees – a change of perspective may be a very useful challenge. We have mentioned that it is important for clinical supervision to sustain boundaries. After a time it may become evident that the parties have blurred the boundaries and are uncertain whether they are friends or colleagues, or in some other relationship that may be beneficial but is no longer what they contracted to be. Self-awareness by both parties should help to monitor this and ensure that, if it occurs, it is used as a marker for change. Length of time could be a very wise guideline in the review process. Clinical supervision relationships do not have a defined 'shelf life' but monitoring whether there should be a change is necessary. Some organisations have a sort of rota system where everyone moves round after two years. Because it is known from the outset that this is the process, it causes no heartache.

Note your thoughts about 'shelf life' for working with another person.

✐ **Your thoughts**

Do you think there is a 'shelf life' for working with other people?

What about afterwards? Boundary issues are important here. Parties may revert to colleagueship, if the supervision was provided internally. If it was provided externally, it may mean the parties will rarely cross paths again. In both cases, but especially in the former, keeping the boundary matters. It would not be appropriate to discuss the new supervisor/supervisee with the previous ones, nor to compare old and new, as this could be de-skilling for all.

In general, then, bringing the supervisory relationship to an ethical ending should mirror the ethical ending aimed for with patients, clients, and those who were close to them.

Conclusion

We end this chapter, and the book, by repeating some of the points made by the UKCC (now the NMC) in its support for clinical supervision:

- Clinical supervision is 'an important part of clinical governance and in the interests of maintaining and improving standards of patient and client care'.
- Clinical supervision supports practice.
- Clinical supervision is a practice-focused professional relationship.
- Ground rules should be agreed so that the supervisor and supervisee approach clinical supervision openly, confidently and with awareness of what is involved.
- Every practitioner should have access to clinical supervision.
- Each supervisor should supervise a reasonable number of practitioners.

A witness statement given by a Marie Curie nurse for this book perhaps sums up what we have endeavoured to show:

👁 **Witness statement**

Although I know that my work is worthwhile, it often tires me, and of course it is often heart-breaking. I sometimes get to a low ebb and then I wonder whether I'm good enough for such a demanding role and I begin to question everything I do – even simple things like changing a bed! Clinical supervision has helped me to see these doubts as a positive. It is *good*, not defeatist, to question your practice and to feel safe in doing that. I appreciate the chance to moan a bit – don't we all! – but I appreciate much more the way it helps me evaluate as well as value what I do.

References

Carroll M (1996) *Counselling Supervision: Theory, Skills and Practice.* Cassell, London

Gibbs G (1988) *Learning by Doing: A Guide to Teaching and Learning Methods.* Further Education Unit, Oxford Brookes University, Oxford

Johns C (1994) Guided reflection. In: Palmer A, Burns S, Bulman C (eds) *Reflective Practice in Nursing. The Growth of the Professional Practitioner.* Blackwell Science, Oxford

Addendum to Chapter Seven

Framework for structured reflection

This framework was adapted from Mezirow J (1981) A critical theory of adult learning and education. *Adult Education* **32**: 3–24. It helps to focus thoughts about critical issues and practice issues which require decision making.

The reflective framework

The experience	Describe the experience or clarify the decision to be made.
The causative factors	Describe the essential factors which contributed to this situation.
The context	Describe the background factors surrounding the situation.
Reflections	How did I feel? How did the patient feel? How did I know? What knowledge affected my decision?
Alternative actions	What choices did I have? What could have been the consequences of these actions?
Emotional impact	What was the emotional impact on the patient, the relatives, self and colleagues?
Learning	Could I have dealt with the situation better? How? What have I learned? Do I need to produce a personal action plan?

Methods of record making

Method one

These sheets are taken from a nurse tutor's log book.

Feb 10 tutorial with 3rd year student (30 mins)

Content	Process and skills
J behind with work, came with many excuses, some valid	Gave good attention Suspended my irritation Listened and paraphrased
What help did she want from me?	Used you-me talk to challenge her to share responsibility for planning her work
Saw me as authority	Goal planning and strategies for avoiding social diversions
Made contract for work for this week	Felt we had a better relationship after challenging her

I need to feel more confident about challenging

Feb 18 Discussion with colleague

Content	Process and skills
Home problems	Moved from coffee bar into her room
Son in trouble	Anxious because I knew I only had 15 minutes before lecture - said so
She angry and frightened	Listened, reflected, and helped her express some feelings
Very tense holding emotions	Helped her to relax to find strength to cope with afternoon

Important others not know

Offered further support later. Felt I had managed the time by not ignoring the limits as I sometimes do - and then feel guilty at rushed ending. How do I manage later if she wants a lot of time? Should I suggest other help? Who?

Feb 21 Staff meeting

Content	Process and skills
Much aggression over forthcoming changes from some of the group Nobody listens to anybody	Tried to use paraphrasing and reflecting to clarify what was happening in the group but got involved and forgot skills Felt very frustrated and angry especially with S — why her?

How can I learn to observe and not get over-involved so that I forget to use my skills - and how can I express my anger without getting upset?

Method two

This supervisee kept a diary for several weeks of interpersonal encounters in his work. He was methodical and creative, so coded some items for quick recording. You might like to attempt something like this yourself. The table below shows his code, which he used at the top of every sheet.

Heading	Explanation	Symbol
Atmosphere	A combination of pressure of time, personal stress and ecological conditions	Poor Good
Setting	Formal/informal Sitting (organised) or other (ie. standing)	F/I
Congruence	(perceived) level of mutual regard/understanding/acceptance	5 is high/1 is low

Here are some examples from his recordings.

Date	Atmosphere	Setting	Person	Work relationship	Congruence
9 Oct	☀	F 🧍	MQ	*Cleaner*	2/3

MQ the centre cleaner was leaving us. I knew she was concerned that she would have to work her notice. She wouldn't normally say so - she's very shy of pushing her own point of view and she sees me very much as the 'boss'. I practised active listening skills and she talked more openly, eventually broaching the subject of working her notice: 'I'll have to work my notice, I know that...'.

I asked her if that is what she wanted to do. Eventually she felt secure enough to say 'No'. Discussed practical problems and agreed the hospice could manage for a week. She seemed relieved and I felt I hadn't imposed my views or the hospice's needs on her - I think the slightest nudge from me and she would have worked her notice in full, causing herself severe personal difficulties.

Note: In retrospect, if I had adopted a similar approach from the out set she would have probably responded more positively to me throughout our relationship - I think she felt before all my concern was for the hospice, not for her as an individual.

Date	Atmosphere	Setting	Person	Work relationship	Congruence
14 Oct	☁	I 🧍	3 members L, P, B	*Colleagues*	3/4

Talking to three team members after a management committee meeting where they had not spoken. Started asking them questions and then consciously paraphrased and reflected - they opened up a lot, spoke of fear and frustration at the meeting - I thought they had just been bored.
Note: when I remember to use AL [active listening] skills I can alter how others relate to me.

Index

The abbreviation CS is used for clinical supervision.

A

absenteeism 37–9
accountable practice 11–12
active listening 64–7
antidiscrimination 54
Aristotle 92
assisted dying 10

B

benefits of CS *see* functions of CS
Bi-Lateral Process Model 104–8
boundary issues 58–9, 128, 129
Bowlby, J 29
British Association for Counselling and Psychotherapy 9, 59

C

Carroll, M 9
challenge 24–5, 63, 69–73, 110–11
    see also feedback
changing supervisors 71, 90, 127–9
clients
    continuity of care 39
    role in CS 5, 82, 95, 100
clinical governance 40–1, 43
Clinical Rhombus Model 99–103
codes of practice 9, 59–60, 125–6
communication skills 62–7
competence levels in supervisees 85–90, 94, 127

confidentiality 50, 54, 58, 59–60, 122–3, 126
conflict (with colleagues) 14, 44–7, 60
continuing professional development 5–8, 42, 122
continuity of care 39
contracts for CS meetings 4, 55, 57–61, 79–81, 119
counselling 2, 67

D

Dass, R 30
data protection 122–3
definitions
    clinical governance 40
    clinical supervision 1–5, 41
    palliative care 91
disciplinary proceedings 117–18
documentation *see* record taking
Double-Helix Model 112
'driver' questionnaire 32–3

E

economic issues
    as cause of conflict 45–6
    sickness rates 37–8
Egan, G 70–1
ego states in TA 104–5
empathy 66–7
ending a working alliance 90, 127–9
ethical issues 9–10, 59–60, 124–7
ethnic minorities 54
exploratory meetings 28, 55, 57–61, 80

F

feedback 12–13, 23–4, 60–1, 73–4
  see also challenge
feedback forms 11
finance
  as cause of conflict 45–6
  sickness rates 37–8
*First Class Service: Quality in the
new NHS* (DoH, 1998a) 43
fitness for work 13, 38
formative function 5–8, 24–5, 60,
  72
functions of CS
  organisational 36–47
  personal 5–16, 35, 129–30
  your thoughts on 61, 70, 72,
  126

G

game-playing in TA 106
generosity 22–3
Gibbs model of recording 120–1
group supervision models 48–9,
  50, 58, 124

H

help-giving 62–3
Holloway Model 113
honesty
  in supervisees 29–30
  in supervisors 26, 73–4
hostility to CS 1, 26, 54, 55–6
'housekeeping' details 57, 58, 80
humanity 25

I

implementation of CS 3–4, 54

J

job satisfaction 13, 36–9
Johari window 34

K

Kübler-Ross, E 111, 118

L

learning 5–8, 24–5, 28–9, 42, 122
line management 3, 53–4
listening skills 63–7

M

malpractice 54, 69, 117–18
Minnesota Job Satisfaction Scale
  36
models
  record-keeping 120–1, 131
  supervision grouping models
  47–50, 79, 93, 124
  supervision process models
  93–113
multi-disciplinary teams 14–15,
  41–7
mutual nature of the CS
relationship 2, 59, 60, 71, 80

N

negative feelings about CS 1, 26,
  54, 55–6
network supervision model 49,
  50, 124
non-hierarchical nature of CS 3,
  53–4
non-judgemental behaviour 25,
  66–7
normative function 8–12, 25–7,
  40–1, 59, 72

structured reflection model 120–1, 131

supervisees
attitudes towards CS 3, 26, 54, 55–6, 84–5
levels of competence 85–90, 94, 127
making the contract 79–81
preparing for the CS meeting 82–4, 119
qualities needed 27–33
relationship with supervisor 2–4, 53–5, 77, 96–7, 127–8
requirements from CS 77–9, 81
responsibilities 29–30, 33, 58, 82–3, 126–7
role in process models of CS 94–7, 100, 103, 107

supervisors
making the contract 57–61
managing group discussions 46–7
qualities needed 19–27
relationship with supervisee 2–4, 53–5, 77, 96–7, 128
responsibilities 27, 58, 126–7
role in process models of CS 97, 99–100, 102–3, 107
skills needed 55, 61–76, 88–90

support 70, 73

T

targets 10–11, 42
Team Development Manual (Woodcock) 44
team work 14–15, 41–7
therapeutic use of self 31
thought-provoking behaviour *see* challenge
time management 4, 22–3, 58

training 5–8, 42, 122
Transactional Analysis (TA) Model 104–8
triad supervision model 49, 50, 74
trust 27, 54–5, 67–9, 83

U

uncompromising behaviour 25–7
United Kingdom Central Council for Nursing, Midwifery and Health Visiting (UKCC) *see* Nursing and Midwifery Council

W

White Paper: The new NHS: modern, dependable (DoH, 1997) 42
work–life balance 13, 30–1
Working Together, Securing a Quality Workforce for the NHS (DoH, 1998b) 43